EXCITING NEWS ABOUT CURES, CONTROLS, AND ALTERNATIVE TREATMENTS

DISCOVER:

- New asthma drugs with the power of steroids . . . but without the side effects
- Help for apnea and nighttime asthma—the dangers that strike while you sleep
- Tips to stop the worst allergy trigger hidden *in your home*
- Better lung function from an inexpensive vitamin supplement
- The best exercise to improve cardiovascular functioning and quality of life
- What you can buy over the counter for real relief
- Echinacea, goldenseal, ginger, and other healing herbs—do they really work?
- The "Flutter"—the Swiss invention that might work wonders for you
- Ancient disciplines now found to offer breathing breakthroughs

and more in . . .

BREATHE RIGHT NOW

Breathe Right
now

**A comprehensive guide to
understanding and treating the
most common breathing disorders**

Laurence A. Smolley, M.D., and
Debra Fulghum Bruce

FOREWORD BY ROB MUZZIO, OLYMPIC DECATHLETE

A Dell Book

Published by
Dell Publishing
a division of
Random House, Inc.
1540 Broadway
New York, New York 10036

ISBN: 0-440-23459-X

Reprinted by arrangement with W. W. Norton & Company, Inc.

Printed in the United States of America

Published simultaneously in Canada

March 1999

10 9 8 7 6 5 4 3 2 1
WCD

To our faithful support team
Martha Handler Smolley
Robert G. Bruce, Jr., M.Div.

Contents

PART 3 Mind over Breath

Foreword

It was a hot summer day in June at the Los Angeles Coliseum, and I was in the biggest competition of my life—the 1984 U.S. Olympic Trials. With the highest decathlon score in the United States in 1984, I was considered a favorite to make the team. Just three weeks earlier I had broken the NCAA decathlon record to become George Mason University's first NCAA champion. At nineteen, I was prepared to be an olympian.

After the first day of the decathlon, I was right on target with my point score to make the team. Instead, I collapsed breathlessly on the track, suffering one of the worst asthma attacks of my life. Rather than earning a trip to the Olympics in 1984, I was immediately taken to the hospital.

This asthma attack should not have surprised me because my asthma began when I was seven. It began late one night when I woke up my parents by coughing, wheezing, and gasping for air. In a panic, we rushed to the emergency room. My parents questioned whether I could breathe long enough to make it to the hospital. The emergency room doctors got my breathing under control by giving me a shot of epinephrine, then told my parents that I had asthma.

The next step my parents took was a visit to my pediatrician, Dr. Richard Evans, who specialized in treating asthma. He had me allergy tested and found I was allergic to just about everything—cats, dogs, certain trees, grasses, molds, feathers, and dust. I remember one of the most traumatic moments of my childhood was having to give our cats away. It took one year to get the cat dander out of our home. Dr. Evans put me on desensitization shots and certain medications to control my asthma. He also told my parents to encourage me to participate in sports, as the more physically fit I became from exercise, the better I would be able to breathe. My father spent time teaching me relaxation drills to help me stay calm, because he knew that if you get excited and tense up, you can make an attack even worse. I had my asthma under control by doing three things:

Seeing my doctor regularly

Taking my medications

Avoiding the things (allergens) that I was allergic to and that might trigger an asthma attack

When I was young and lived at home, my asthma stayed under control. The real problems began when I moved out of my house and went to college. I gradually stopped taking my medications and seeing my doctor. Foolishly, as a young adult, I went in and out of a state of denial about having asthma. When I would have an attack, I would think that I was supposed to suffer and that is why they call it an asthma attack. Unfortunately, I continued to believe this, suffering frequent asthma attacks until 1991.

In 1991, I made the World Championship team and was ranked third in the United States. While I was at the

World Championships in Tokyo, Japan, I developed a cough that the doctor labeled bronchitis. Of course, I didn't fare too well in the competition. When I came home, I was over the bronchitis and ready to train for the 1992 Olympic Games. However, each time I went out for a run, I had to stop after five minutes because of difficulty breathing during asthma attacks. This upset my wife, Natalie, who said, "Rob, this is crazy! You are trying to compete against the greatest athletes in the world, and you cannot even jog for five minutes. There must be something you can do."

After much encouragement from my wife, I finally went to see Dr. Donna Schuster, an asthma and allergy specialist, in November 1991. When I told Dr. Schuster I wanted to make the 1992 Olympic team, she said although there wasn't much time, I could get my asthma under control if I followed her management plan.

The first thing she did was perform a simple lung function evaluation called spirometry. She found that I could exhale only 36 percent of the volume of air expected of a normal person my age, weight, and height and explained this was the reason I could not run for more than five minutes at a time. Dr. Schuster said this meant I had inflammation in my bronchial tubes, and the inflammation was the origin of my breathing problems. In people with moderate to severe asthma, the key to controlling the disease and leading a normal life is reducing the inflammation. This was the beginning of my asthma education.

Dr. Schuster put me on a combination of medications, including an inhaled bronchodilator called albuterol (Proventil or Ventolin are the brand names used), which relaxes the muscles in the walls of the bronchial tubes to keep them wide open, and an inhaled corticosteroid called triamcinolone (Azmacort is the brand name used) to reduce the inflammation. To be honest, it was the inhaled corticosteroid that turned my life around as it began to control the inflammation. I now take these medicines several times a day, every day, and call my medication routine my "recipe." I've learned that as long as I stick to this, I don't have any problems with my asthma.

Before starting my "recipe," I would miss as many as ten to twenty practices a year due to asthma. Once I stayed with the medication regime and got my asthma under control, I missed no more practices because of asthma. My life had been changed unbelievably, and I no longer feared asthma and its effects on my performance. I learned that when I had problems with my asthma, it was because I was being *reactive*, trying to stop an attack once it had begun. To control asthma, you must be *proactive* and prevent an attack from even starting. This is where the inhaled corticosteroid made the biggest difference, controlling the inflammation before it could build up and cause an attack.

Once I realized that asthma was not going to go away, I had to improve the quality of my life by keeping my asthma under control. What is most important, I achieved my lifelong dream of competing for the United States in the Olympics. I will never forget placing fifth at the Summer Olympic Games in Barcelona, Spain! I know that if I had continued to have frequent asthma attacks, I would have *never* made the team.

A most powerful influence has been the support of my family. When I was young, it was my parents who helped me control this disease. Now, my wife has convinced me that I don't have to suffer with shortness of breath and wheezing anymore. I realize now why it is so important to make a positive impact on the people in our lives who have asthma.

I know that asthma can be a frightening disease when uncontrolled. If you don't control your asthma, it will control you and may even threaten your life. It does not matter what your occupation is, whether you are an athlete, writer, teacher, painter, doctor, musician, or magician. Asthma recognizes no barriers. It will beat you down . . . if you don't control it.

Since I have been through the bad times, I now share pieces of my life with people in hopes they will not have to go through what I have. Educating yourself about this disease is the best way to beat it. Many people ignore their symptoms; many people don't even know that they have it.

Asthma is just one example of a respiratory disease that may adversely affect your life. Knowledge can lead to proper appreciation that a problem exists and that specific help is available. Whether you have asthma, allergy, sinusitis, emphysema, or other respiratory problems, I urge everyone to read this book. You can help yourself or someone you love to enjoy a normal, higher quality of life. It is possible to alleviate the unnecessary coughing, congestion, wheezing, shortness of breath, panic, fear, and deaths due to respiratory diseases that can be successfully managed.

Rob Muzzio
Olympic decathlete

Acknowledgments

In our quest to provide accurate and up-to-date information on respiratory problems we have sought and received generous assistance from a gifted and select group of health care professionals. We express our gratitude to them all.

James K. Stoller, M.D.; head, Section of Respiratory Therapy, Department of Pulmonary and Critical Care Medicine, Cleveland Clinic Foundation, Cleveland, Ohio (alpha-1 antitrypsin deficiency and emphysema)

Prasoon Jain, M.D., and Joseph A. Golish, M.D.; Department of Pulmonary and Critical Care Medicine, Cleveland Clinic Foundation, Cleveland, Ohio (asthma)

Jerry O. Ciocon, M.D.; Chief, Section of Geriatrics, Cleveland Clinic Florida, Fort Lauderdale, Florida (breathing problems of the elderly)

Jeffrey C. Wolkowicz, M.D.; chairman, Department of Pulmonary Diseases, Cleveland Clinic Florida, Fort

Lauderdale, Florida (chronic obstructive pulmonary disease and sinobronchial syndrome)

Islon Woolf, M.D.; chief medical resident, Department of Medicine, Cleveland Clinic Florida, Fort Lauderdale, Florida (chiropractic and acupuncture for respiratory problems)

Ian Nathanson, M.D.; pediatric pulmonologist, physician-in-chief, Nemour's Children's Clinic, Orlando, Florida (breathing problems in newborn and young children)

Sean R. Muldoon, M.D.; pulmonologist, private practice, Jacksonville, Florida (occupational asthma)

Philip Hardy, M.D.; orthopedist, private practice, Jacksonville, Florida (exercise and respiratory disease)

Karen E. Malcolm, Pharm.D.; University of Florida, Jacksonville, Florida (drug therapy of respiratory disease)

Paul Wubbena, M.D.; private practice, Jacksonville, Florida (allergy, asthma, and immunology)

Frank Novakoski, M.S.; Jacksonville, Florida (exercise physiology)

Allan Decker, M.A.; private practice, Jacksonville, Florida (stress management)

April Dodd, D.C., and Daniel Dodd, D.C.; chiropractors, private practice, Jacksonville, Florida (chiropractic and complementary therapies)

Nicholas Hall, Ph.D.; director, Institute for Health and Human Performance, Orlando, Florida (psychoneuroimmunology)

Harris H. McIlwain, M.D.; rheumatologist and gerontologist, private practice, Tampa, Florida (geriatric concerns)

Lori Steinmeyer, M.S.; R.D./L.D., Tampa, Florida (nutrition)

Patrick Malone, director, Massage Therapy Associates, Chicago, Illinois (therapeutic touch)

A special thanks goes to Rob Muzzio, Olympic decathlete, for his inspirational story about how he overcame the obstacles of respiratory disease to place fifth in the Summer Olympic Games in Barcelona, Spain.

We also appreciate the excellent skills of Irys Caristo of the Cleveland Clinic Florida who helped communication to continually flow between the authors during the writing of this book.

We are grateful to our editor, Gerald Howard, for his guidance, excellent editing skills, and enthusiasm for this project.

Breathe Right
now

Introduction:
New Hope for
Better Breathing

Everyone has experienced breathing difficulties from time to time. For some people, these symptoms subside, and they can move on with their lives. But for millions who suffer daily with breathing disorders, such debilitating symptoms as coughing, sneezing, stuffy nose, breathlessness, and wheezing are relentless and cause poor quality of life. Many claim that breathing problems have ruined much of their lives. You deserve to know that with today's treatment options; it does *not* have to be that way.

Perhaps you are thinking, "This book will not help me. My nose is constantly congested and just thinking about exercise causes shortness of breath." Well, we have good news! We have experienced all types of respiratory disorders, both professionally and personally. As a pulmonologist and sleep disorders specialist, Dr. Smolley's professional experience in treating respiratory diseases for the past sixteen years keeps him acutely aware of breakthroughs in diagnosis and treatment. Debra Fulghum Bruce has a strong genetic link in her family to allergy, sinusitis, asthma, and chronic obstructive pulmonary disease (COPD), with every member in her immediate and extended family suffering from some type of respiratory symptom daily. It is her personal challenge to find answers to help those closest to her.

Dr. Laurence Smolley

In medical school and during my internship-residency training, I enjoyed learning about all the various specialties of medicine. I particularly treasured the time spent in the "Chest" building at the Kings County Hospital in Brooklyn, New York, where I helped care for patients with the whole gamut of respiratory diseases. My supervising physicians were excellent role models, and I admired them very much.

However, the reason that I chose to apply for a fellowship in pulmonary diseases was because of a tragic personal experience. One summer when I was home from college, my father died right before my eyes during a sudden attack of shortness of breath. Clumsy resuscitative attempts did not work, and the paramedics from 911 in New York City arrived far too late. I know my father died an early death at age fifty-nine, because he ignored the warning signs and symptoms of disease. Perhaps if he knew more and sought treatment earlier, he would still be alive today.

The symptom of shortness of breath, along with a host of other breathing difficulties, has intrigued me over the years. Figuring out the exact cause of the problem is essential before proper treatment can be applied. My experience dealing with patients with respiratory diseases has shown me that those who are best informed and take an active role in their medical care generally have fewer hospitalizations and longer lifespans.

I know that the treatment choices in this book really do work. These options have helped thousands of sufferers across the country regain the ability to breathe clearly, and, thus, improve quality of life.

Debra Fulghum Bruce

My experience with respiratory diseases is very personal and serves as motivation for writing this book. As a child, I grew up thinking that nasal congestion, sinus drainage, and coughing on arising or during exercise were normal. After all, no one in my family could breathe well, suffering as they did from both allergy and asthma, so these symptoms were all I knew. Even as young as five years old, I was given a cup of strong coffee on awakening to help open clogged airways. On school days, my mother would warn, "Don't run at recess if you have trouble breathing."

Although I was oblivious to our family history, I vaguely remember my parents talking about my paternal grandfather who had bronchiectasis, an older cousin who died of complications of asthma, an aunt who suffered with emphysema, and several relatives on my mother's side who had constant headaches from chronic sinusitis. When I got a cold and had to stay home because of "funny whistles in my chest (bronchial asthma)," again, I figured this was "normal." You will learn in this book that these symptoms are not "normal," and there is treatment!

After I was married (to a man who had childhood asthma) and our third child, Ashley, was born, I was forced to begin a personal quest for answers to better breathing. Ashley had fluid in her ears the first year of life, along with a host of skin allergies. During the preschool years, she began to have frequent bouts of bronchitis and sinusitis. At age seven, after a lengthy bout of the flu and bronchitis, Ashley went through allergy testing and was diagnosed with many allergies and chronic asthma. She was not alone: our older children, Rob and Brittnye, were also diagnosed with allergies and asthma and suffered daily from symptoms of nasal congestion, coughing, or wheezing.

It was at a family reunion that I realized someone had to take immediate action to find relief for our strong genetic predisposition to breathing problems. While sitting with a group of relatives, I will never forget how several aunts, uncles, and cousins took puffs from asthma inhalers to open swollen airways. Conversation centered on who had tried the latest nonsedating antihistamines or who had found relief for sinus pain and pressure. Later that evening, I felt hopeless as I surveyed our family's medicine closet. It was filled with inhaler boxes and canisters, bottles of over-the-counter decongestants and antihistamines, prescription antibiotics, and steroid nasal sprays, to mention just a few.

Today, I know there is hope. Through regular visits with our allergist, talking with many health care professionals across the country, and doing years of research, I have realized that everyone deserves the opportunity to breathe right now. No matter what respiratory problems you face, we will show you a wealth of available treatments that will allow you to have the highest quality of life, including exercise. And the best way to better breathing is to educate yourself about the problem, then work as a team with your physician and your family using the proactive steps as outlined in this book.

We've Found the Answers

We wrote this book to offer new hope to those who wake up each day struggling for breath and are frustrated through the day when breathlessness occurs with minimal exertion. Throughout this book, you will learn how some of the country's finest health care professionals treat breathing disorders with both conventional medicine and complementary methods such as biofeedback or acupuncture. You will find accurate descriptions and explanations of the most common breathing problems and learn the latest, most effective methods for diagnosis, treatment, and prevention.

Because almost everyone who suffers from one breathing problem is likely to have others, we have written the first book that covers most common breathing disorders. For example, you may suffer with allergy and asthma and then develop emphysema or chronic bronchitis from smoking. To breathe optimally, you must recognize the specific diseases and promptly seek prevention and treatment measures that are likely to be effective.

As you identify your particular problem, it is important to realize that you are not alone. An estimated 60 million people in the United States today have allergy and asthma. Another 20 million suffer with chronic lung disease. These problems are very common and know no barriers of race, sex, or age. Allergy and asthma alone account for one out of nine trips to the doctor; children also figure high in this number as breathing problems account for more than one out of every five trips to the pediatrician.

Breathing problems are nothing new to millions. However, most people remain unaware of how these diseases which cause shortness of breath, chronic cough, wheezing, and difficulty performing the activities of daily living can be controlled. Must those with breathing disorders simply accept the feeling of choking or strangling? Should they tolerate the limited mobility, inability to exercise, or sleepless nights that often accompany nocturnal breathlessness? The answer is *no!*

Allergic Triggers

Some believe that it is only children, the elderly, or smokers who suffer breathing problems, but that is not true. Breathing problems can begin in the first year of life. Or, some people can be disease-free until retirement age and then be faced with shortness of breath from COPD, or adult-onset asthma. Allergies can come and go. This means you may be allergic to a certain food such as peanuts, soy, or eggs as a young child and then during your teen years develop an allergy to pollen, mold, or that favorite down comforter.

Some triggers of allergy and asthma include pregnancy (from hormonal and blood-flow changes), viral infection such as cold or flu, exposure to something in the environment, and food. Food allergies can be fatal. A recent report from the National Institutes of Health (NIH) estimates that more than 1 million people a year suffer from a life-threatening anaphylactic reaction to food. Anaphylaxis is the most severe form of allergy and involves the entire body. When it occurs, the blood pressure plunges to dangerously low levels. There is also swelling throughout the body. When this occurs in the walls of the bronchial tubes, there may be a severe obstruction which slows down the exit of air from the lungs. When this occurs in the larynx or upper airway, air may not be able to enter the lungs.

More recently, scientists have found that estrogen levels trigger asthma in some women. Women with asthma may experience a worsening of symptoms, including increased coughing and wheezing, during the week before menstruation. These new findings were reported at the 1996 American College of Clinical Pharmacy by researcher Mary Chandler, an associate professor of pharmacy at the University of Kentucky, who followed fourteen women for three menstrual cycles. These women kept careful records of their asthma symptoms and measured their airflows with peak expiratory flow meters (PEFRs) (more on this indispensable tool for asthma management in Chapter 4).

Determined by symptoms, and also the peak flow rate, all fourteen women in the study experienced at least a 20 percent increase in symptoms during the premenstrual phase. Researchers found that asthma symptoms were mildest on day 13 of the cycle and strongest at day 26, when estrogen is at its lowest level.

Emotions also influence some breathing problems. In fact, it used to be thought that asthma was a psychosomatic disease. Now we know that stress may be a trigger. In other words, if you don't have asthma, emotional stress cannot cause it. However, if you do have asthma, being upset, crying, or getting angry can worsen the symptoms or even bring on an attack.

Predisposition

Although factors such as respiratory infections, air pollution, diet, and emotional makeup play key roles in precipitating problems, your genetic heritage is also important as Debra shared in her personal story. For example, if one parent has allergies, each child has a one-in-three chance of also having allergies. If both parents suffered from allergy, the probability that each child may also suffer is close to 100 percent. Family history also appears to predispose you to asthma and COPD, with three-fifths of all asthma cases being hereditary.

A Holistic Approach

Obviously many risk factors play key roles in breathing disorders, including genetics, diet, illnesses, hormones, environment, and emotional makeup. Because of this crucial mind-body interplay, you deserve to know that taking a holistic, or comprehensive, approach to better breathing can offer even greater benefit. This book will take that approach and explain the importance of:

Understanding risk factors and learning how to reduce your risk

Getting an accurate diagnosis using the latest diagnostic tools

Developing a management plan with your doctor and family

Knowing which medications are best to treat and prevent your particular symptoms

Understanding and avoiding the triggers of your breathing disorder

Exercising to maximize aerobic fitness by conditioning the heart and other muscles

Preventing exercise-induced breathing problems

Reducing stress

Eating nutritional foods to maximize immune defenses against infections

Using healing foods filled with phytochemicals, antioxidants, and flavonoids

Maintaining a normal weight

Obtaining restful sleep, even with nocturnal breathing problems

A Comprehensive Guide

No matter what problem you have, the goal should be to reach the stage at which the disorder can be controlled. Once this is accomplished, returning to normal activity and exercise is possible. There will be improved sleep and a greater sense of well-being. Although we outline a broad spectrum of treatments throughout the book, we continually emphasize the importance of preventive measures to *avoid* acute attacks and *control* chronic problems.

While this book is not meant to be an exhaustive medical reference on respiratory diseases, it is a comprehensive guide book to help you breathe better. To gain further insight about your particular problem, call the support groups listed and check the web sites offered on the Internet. If you have any questions about your breathing disorder, we encourage you to write these down and ask your health care professional.

In short, the main ingredient in the treatment and prevention of breathing disorders is you—*if* you begin a comprehensive program to eliminate risk factors, boost your immune power, and stay healthy despite your chronic condition. In other words, you can change things in your life so that the chances of your problems worsening are greatly reduced. You can begin to live your life again and move from patient to person—to happier times at home and improved quality times at work and play—without the constant fear of shortness of breath.

Let's get started.

Part 1

An Introduction to Breathing Problems

chapter 1

The Fire of Life: How We Breathe

After a springtime bout with the flu, Sam coughed day and night for weeks. When summer arrived, he was still coughing and thought it was the result of a mold allergy due to the summer rainy season. Again, Sam ignored the cough. Fall came and Sam was still coughing. At that time, this thirty-seven-year-old man mentally wrote it off as a "temporary allergy to the change of temperatures." It wasn't until he was raking the leaves one brisk November day that Sam knew he was in trouble. After working vigorously in the cold outdoors, he literally could not catch his breath.

Fortunately his family physician had an office less than a mile away from his home. There, Sam's doctor took his medical history, ran several diagnostic tests to see whether there was an obstruction in his airflow, and diagnosed him with cough-variant asthma. This is a type of asthma in which coughing is the main symptom instead of wheezing. To eliminate the cough, chest tightness, and congestion, the doctor gave Sam newer inhaled medications. These helped to relax the tight airways, reduce inflammation, control the cough, and prevent dangerous episodes of shortness of breath.

When a specific breathing problem appears, aren't many of us, like Sam, reluctant to call a physician, hoping it will go away on its own? Julia, a forty-two-year-old preschool teacher, thought the constant, thick drainage down the back of her throat was the remnant of a cold. It wasn't until she woke up several mornings later with a fever accompanied by throbbing pain in her head, jaws, and teeth that she sought a diagnosis. The verdict? An acute sinus infection that needed antibiotic treatment and decongestants. Repeatedly, many people seek medical intervention only after they have harbored symptoms for weeks to months. Often by the time the medications are started, damage has occurred that takes even more time to heal.

It is important to understand that an accurate diagnosis is important before you can treat and prevent breathing problems. Each of us is different. The specific medication and treatment program that works for a family member, friend, or the convincing actor on the decongestant commercial may *not* be the correct one for your problem.

Respiratory diseases include many disorders that affect one or more of the parts of the respiratory system. It is difficult to understand respiratory problems without a clear and thorough understanding of how breathing works. Let's review how we breathe, the problems that may interrupt this process, and the latest treatment methods.

The Normal Respiratory System

Respiration is a basic process of life. It is through this process that we get energy for growth and activity. For life to go on in most animals, continuous energy is required. Many years ago, oxygen was recognized as the gas required to maintain the "fire of life" in animals. In fact, it was once believed that the heart was the internal furnace where the "fire of life" kept the blood boiling.

Today we know differently. We know that each cell (the smallest living animal unit) has minute structures called *mitochondria* where the oxidation of food takes place. *Oxidation* is the combination of oxygen with the carbon and hydrogen atoms that make up food matter such as carbohydrates. During this process, energy is released that is used to drive the various life-supporting functions inside the cell. Although cells have other ways of meeting their energy needs, they are inefficient. Eventually the cell must go back to using oxygen.

Oxygen and carbohydrates are convenient sources for meeting the energy requirements of cells in living creatures. The oxygen in the atmosphere is continuously replenished by the plants that surround us, especially by the algae in the oceans. Using the sun's radiant energy, plants take carbon and make carbohydrates through *photosynthesis*. The process of photosynthesis produces oxygen which is then released into the air. So, animals and plants make up a cooperative system with two gases, oxygen and carbon dioxide, exchanged in an ongoing cycle driven by the sun's energy.

The Lungs

How do we get this oxygen into our bodies? This is one main function of our lungs. They get oxygen from the air into the bloodstream and allow carbon dioxide to escape from the body. Although the lungs are the main part of the respiratory system, the nose, throat, trachea, chest wall, and certain muscles, such as the diaphragm, also play important roles in breathing (see Figure 1.1).

Parts of the brain and nervous system are involved with the control of the size of the breaths and the frequency of breathing. The *autonomic nervous system* is the part that regulates the organs in the body over which we have no voluntary control. This system consists of two branches:

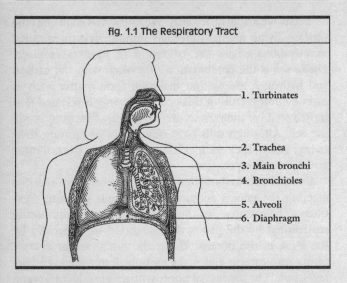

fig. 1.1 The Respiratory Tract

1. Turbinates
2. Trachea
3. Main bronchi
4. Bronchioles
5. Alveoli
6. Diaphragm

the *sympathetic* and the *parasympathetic* nervous systems. In an asthma attack, triggering the sympathetic branch causes airways to expand, or dilate. Stimulating the parasympathetic branch results in *bronchoconstriction*, or constriction of the airways.

The way in which parts of the brain and nervous system work together to produce breathing patterns is very complex and depends on the levels of oxygen and carbon dioxide in the blood. Other factors also affect breathing patterns such as whether we are awake or asleep, have pain or anxiety, are overweight, or have some disease that throws off the normal balance of acid in our body.

The Nose

If you have constant nasal congestion due to allergies or hay fever, you may argue this fact, but most normal adults breathe mainly through the nose. Oxygen-rich air enters the nose and mouth where it is warmed and mixed with water vapor in the upper respiratory passages.

The function of the nose besides providing for the sense of smell is to protect the lower airway from cold or contaminated air. The air we breathe varies in temperature, humidity, and purity. This air temperature is adjusted close to body temperature during its passage through the nose; simultaneously, air is properly humidified, or moisturized, and particles in the air are filtered out.

The openings of the nose, or nostrils, are lined with skin and a thin mesh of hair. This hair projects into the airway to provide the first filter for dust or other particles such as smoke, pollen, and bacteria. The septum divides the inside of the nose into two parts. The left and right nasal chambers have side walls complicated structurally yet very important functionally.

There are four tubular structures called *turbinates* that project into the nasal chambers and increase the surface area of the walls of the inside of the nose. A mucous membrane that is rich in blood vessels covers these turbinates. The turbinates may swell and cause nasal obstruction. This nasal obstruction, which can be caused by a variety of conditions, usually seems worse when you are lying down. This is because the tissue fluids and blood tend to pool in your head when a recumbent position is taken. Sometimes at night while reclining on one side, this side becomes clogged and it is necessary to turn in bed to breathe easily. Then the other side may become obstructed. It may become a vicious cycle that can ruin a restful night's sleep.

The Sinuses

There are small openings in the walls of your nose that communicate with your *sinuses*. The four sinuses developed as outpouchings of the nasal mucous membrane, which is composed of cells. These cells are specialized in that some have cilia and others produce mucus. It's easy to confuse the words *mucous* and *mucus*. Although they sound the same, they have distinct meanings. *Mucous* (adjective) means covered with mucus or containing mucus. The mucous membrane is a soft, pink, skinlike structure, which lines many cavities and tubes in the body, such as the respiratory tract. The mucous membrane secretes a fluid containing *mucus* (noun), a viscid, slippery secretion, which helps to lubricate and protect certain parts of the body.

The entire lining of the nose is covered with a thin coat of moisture made up of mucus. This mucus rests on top of the *cilia* of the cells making up the mucous membrane. Cilia are like tiny hairs that beat or wave rhythmically to carry anything on their surface in the direction of their motion, generally out of the respiratory tract. This is achieved by a rapid beat, with the cilia standing up straight, and a slower phase, with the cilia bending in the opposite direction. The mucus is sticky and collects tiny airborne particles that come into contact with it. This coating also contains enzymes that destroy most bacteria.

About 85 to 90 percent of the tiniest particles, 5 microns (millionths of a meter) in diameter, and larger are blocked and removed in the nose and nasopharynx. Yet, smaller particles may get into the lower respiratory tract. When the action of the mucous coat is altered by trauma, drying, irritating chemicals, or any other factor, the nose, sinuses, and lower respiratory tract become more susceptible to infection.

The Lower Respiratory Tract

Warmed, properly humidified, and filtered, air now passes from the nose and mouth to the larynx, moving past vocal cords to the *trachea*, or main windpipe. The trachea then divides into left and right main bronchi which convey air to the two lungs. These main *bronchi* have cartilage in their walls and are essentially like rigid pipes. The main bronchi are well suited for conducting air down to the smaller bronchi and bronchioles into which they divide like the branches of a tree.

In the *bronchial walls,* there is muscle that may contract in response to various stimuli with resultant constriction of the airway as in asthma. *Bronchioles* divide into even smaller bronchioles that eventually serve as sites of gas exchange. The smallest subdivisions known as *respiratory bronchioles* bud out into *alveolar ducts* and *alveoli.*

Conducting airways deliver fresh air to the alveoli. These airways have a mucous coat similar to that of the nose and sinuses. As in the nose, *mucociliary clearance* removes particles that land on this surface. However, problems in the lungs and in gas exchange may arise when damage occurs to this mucociliary mechanism, either from cigarette smoking or infection.

The *alveoli* are tiny sacs that branch off the smallest airways like clusters of grapes. Alveoli where actual gas exchange occurs are closely surrounded by networks of tiny blood vessels called *capillaries,* which carry blood to pick up oxygen from the freshly inhaled air. At that time, carbon dioxide leaves the blood to enter the alveoli so it can be blown out of the body on exhalation.

The number of breaths per minute and the depth of inhalation are closely controlled by the *central nervous system* through receptors that monitor the levels of oxygen and carbon dioxide in the blood. (The *central nervous system* is the anatomical term for the brain and the spinal cord.) The muscles of respiration provide the forces of inspiration and help with expiration. The contraction of certain muscles enlarges the chest whereas the contraction of other muscle groups compresses it. Expiration is normally an involuntary process dependent on the elastic recoil properties of the expanded chest wall and the lungs themselves.

The Diaphragm

The *diaphragm* separates the chest cavity from the abdomen. It is the main provider of inspiratory muscle force and is called the "second vital pump"; the heart is considered the first. When the diaphragm contracts, it pushes down into the abdomen. Because the diaphragm is attached to the inside of the chest wall, this movement enlarges the chest cavity. When the chest cavity expands, it results in a drop in pressure inside, as compared with the pressure of the atmosphere outside. This lower pressure is transmitted from the lungs to the airways and up to the throat, nose, and mouth. At this time, air is pushed by atmospheric pressure into the upper airways and down through the conducting airways to the alveoli.

Disruption of Breathing

Chances are great that you would have no need for this book *if* your respiratory system functioned efficiently, as explained. However, as you know, normal breathing is frequently disrupted by any process that affects even the smallest part of the respiratory system. For example, if you are allergic to down in a pillow or to dust mites on your bed, you may experience nasal congestion, as discussed on page 17, when you lie down to sleep. The increased resistance to your airflow can cause breathing discomfort, frequent wakening, and even snoring, which disturb your sleep and make you drag through the next day. Similarly, an infection, which causes extra mucus production in the bronchi, may cause difficulty breathing because of blocked airflow. A cold virus may create havoc throughout your entire respiratory system, including such uncomfortable symptoms as sinus congestion and drainage, inflammation in the airways, bronchoconstriction, and wheezing. And, serious diseases, as described in this book, can cause continuing breathing difficulties.

Knowledge Is Crucial

It has long been recognized that when many people with breathing problems are given a diagnosis, much of their anxiety and distress results from a lack of knowledge about the illness. Not only are they frightened by an inability to catch their breath, but their uneasiness about living with a chronic disease is overwhelming. Using the large amount of information given in this book, along with an acute awareness of how your body functions and your specific respiratory symptoms, you will be better equipped to take control of your illness. Control will come from following the medication regime your doctor prescribes to relieve and control respiratory problems, exercising regularly, eating nutritional foods, getting healing sleep, and trying alternative therapies to destress your body. In doing so, you will start on the path to optimal health—even with a chronic respiratory illness—which will greatly enhance your quality of life.

chapter 2

Understanding Allergy and Nasal Disorders

There is an old proverb that states, "Life is in the breath. He who half breathes, half lives." If you suffer from allergies and nasal problems, this proverb is nothing new, as Mac would testify. This thirty-seven-year-old marriage and family counselor claims to know all about half-breathing. After all, he has lived with uncontrolled allergies most of his life. Mac cannot even remember the last time his nasal passages did not feel swollen and stuffy and added, "My allergies are so bad that I can look at springtime flowers in a painting and immediately start sneezing."

Then there are people like Bev, whose nose never feels swollen, just drippy. In fact, she would not know there was a problem except for the constant sinus drip on the back of her throat, twenty-four hours a day, even when she goes to sleep at night. When Bev takes over-the-counter sinus medications, the drip stops. Yet the side effects of nervousness, insomnia, and lack of appetite seem even worse than the illness at times. "I have to decide each day whether I would rather choke on the sinus drainage or feel horrible from the medication."

What happens when you have allergies or nasal problems? Many people tell of living with a constant nasal congestion, pounding sinus headaches, or frequent colds, fevers, scratchy throats, earaches, and infections. In all cases, the symptoms are not only uncomfortable, but they can make you feel downright grouchy.

Forty-year-old Linda, who has had allergies to anything and everything since childhood, found that as she got older, her allergies became more chronic and annoying. Before finding relief with a new prescription steroid inhaler, discussed in Chapter 5, her constantly stuffy and swollen nose caused her to wake up frequently during the night; this made her feel tired and sluggish the next day— and this was on a "good" day.

On the "bad" days, especially for weeks during pollen season, Linda's problems dramatically increased to continual sneezing and thick drainage on the back of her throat. This resulted in hoarseness, a scratchy throat, and increased irritability. Until she sought help, allergy stole from her quality of life and also affected her relationships with family and friends.

Not only are the symptoms of allergy and nasal problems annoying, as Linda experienced, but upper respiratory problems are time consuming and expensive. Have you ever tabulated how much money you spend on breathing medications? The total may surprise you! Approximately $5 billion are spent annually in the United States for medication (over the counter or prescription) for relieving nasal congestion. Although these problems can seem benign at first, they usually result in frequent trips to the doctor. Sometimes costly laboratory tests or X rays may be needed for diagnosis. The side effects of various medications may cause disturbing symptoms, and you may lose valuable days at work or school.

Because the nasal passage is a major entry gate for

viruses and allergens, the nose and sinuses may be associated with many lung disorders. This sinus or nasal passage inflammation may trigger reflexes and produce asthma. Keep in mind that *allergy is the number one cause of asthma*.

So what is the answer? It lies in your hands. While most breathing problems have no *cure*, it is reasonable for you to fully *control* most symptoms using the many treatments available today. Before you can begin to find relief, let's review the common risk factors, symptoms, and diagnostic tests for many types of allergies and nasal disorders.

Allergy

If allergy is your problem, you have a great deal of company. An estimated 60 million Americans suffer from allergies, including skin reactions. Unlike colds and other infections, an overreaction of your immune system to an ordinarily harmless substance causes allergy. If you have allergies, you have a hypersensitivity to substances known as *allergens* which trigger these reactions.

Think back to the last time you suffered from an allergy attack. Your allergic reaction may have been caused by something you ate (corn, wheat, eggs, yeast, soybeans, or medications), the air you breathed (filled with pollen, mold spores, smoke, and pollutants), or the things you touched (wool, latex, or common household cleaning products).

Do you remember how your body reacted? Many people go from breathing normally to suddenly feeling a tickle in their throat, an itchy nose, and unending sneezing. A host of other symptoms soon follow such as swollen nasal passages, headache, drippy, irritated eyes, and even reddened blotchy skin. Who hasn't also experienced such revealing cosmetic signs of allergy as the dark undereye circles that make you look as if you haven't slept in weeks?

What Causes Allergy?

You can probably blame your genes: your inherited genetic makeup can predispose you to allergies. Yet for symptoms to occur, there must also be frequent exposure to allergens, such as dust mites, animals, pollens, or molds, to stimulate the allergic reaction. The problem arises when someone with respiratory allergies meets an allergy trigger, or allergen and a reaction takes place.

Knowledge of three components is important for understanding how allergies happen.

Mast cells These are the allergy-causing cells in the mucous lining of the nose, sinuses, and bronchi that contain chemicals like *histamine*. Histamine is the substance that causes nasal stuffiness and dripping in a cold or hay fever, bronchoconstriction in asthma, and itchy spots in a skin allergy.

Antibodies Antibodies are specific types of proteins called *immunoglobulins,* which are part of the body's defense mechanism. They may attach to a foreign protein in the body. The most important antibody during an allergic reaction is *immunoglobulin E (IgE).* While everyone makes IgE, people who have a genetic predisposition toward an allergy make larger quantities.

Allergens These are substances that trigger the body's allergic reaction. When the IgE on a mast cell combines with an allergen, an allergic reaction may result.

On Guard

The immune system, which is designed to guard and protect the body against invaders, may produce the antibody immunoglobulin E (IgE) if exposed to certain allergens. This IgE antibody, which causes allergy, binds to the surface membrane of the mast cells. Mast cells are found in all tissues of the human body, such as the skin, but especially in the mucous lining of the respiratory system.

Let's assume, for example, that you are allergic to roses. When you smell the fragrant arrangement of roses, the allergens enter your nose or bronchial tubes where they may combine with the IgE on the mast cells. If two IgE antibodies on a mast cell are bridged by the allergen, the cell will then release histamine. This is that powerful chemical most allergic people dread as it causes nasal and bronchial tube tissues to swell because of *vasodilation,* or leaking of plasma and widening of the blood vessels. Histamine also causes bronchial constriction and increased mucus secretion.

So, what is the result of your momentary enjoyment of roses? Miserable symptoms such as a runny nose, sneezing, watery eyes, coughing, and sometimes wheezing. If the reaction occurs in your nose and eyes, you will have allergic rhinitis, or hay fever. If the reaction is in your chest, asthma results with inflammation, cough, wheezing, and mucus production. Red, itchy skin rashes are another result of allergy. Did you ever think that smelling a rose could cause so much chaos in your body?

Immediate or Late Phase

Allergic reactions may be *immediate* or *late phase.* An immediate reaction occurs when you may have contact with an allergen, such as a flower, mold, or mildew, and then have a reaction within fifteen minutes. Or, you may not have any symptoms for hours and then experience a late-phase reaction. Both of these reactions can go away with or without treatment, or they may recur for days, weeks, or months.

A reaction to an allergen results in a specific disease, like allergy, allergic rhinitis, or skin allergy *(allergic der-*

matitis). Therefore, the first step in treating any allergy is to find out which substances or allergens are causing your problem. Through a physical examination, taking your medical history, and doing a series of skin tests to see which allergens react with your system, your doctor can begin to piece the allergy puzzle together. Sometimes your keen observation of what causes the symptoms such as cold air, foods, pollen, dust, perfumes, plants, or animals can help suggest which allergens are responsible for the reactions you feel.

Depending on the type of allergy, your doctor will do specific tests as discussed in Chapter 4. For example, if you have allergic rhinitis (hay fever), your doctor will focus on doing a nasal examination and may look at a sample of mucus under the microscope. If you have asthma, breathing tests such as spirometry (page 69) will be taken to see whether there is an obstruction in your airflow. If your disease is allergic dermatitis, resulting in inflamed and itchy skin or hives, your doctor will focus on specific sensitivity tests to see whether you have reactions.

Common Allergens, Irritants, and Physical Changes That Trigger an Allergic Response

Plant pollens	Medications (aspirin, anti-inflammatory drugs, penicillin, beta blockers)
Tree pollens	
Molds and mildew	
Household dust (dust mites)	Insect stings
Animal dander	Hormones
Industrial chemicals	Smoke
Cockroaches	Perfumes or inhalants
Feathers	Respiratory infections
Foods (chocolate, shellfish, milk, citrus, eggs, nuts, corn)	Gases
	Weather changes
Food additives or colorings (sulfites or preservatives)	Cold air
	Exercise

Allergic Rhinitis

Rhinitis is inflammation or swelling of the mucous membrane of the nose. Allergic rhinitis is the single most common chronic allergic disease experienced by humans and affects more than 40 million people in the United States. It is more commonly known as *hay fever,* a term used when symptoms occur in late summer.

In case you were wondering, your allergic rhinitis, or hay fever, is not caused by hay nor is it accompanied by a fever. It is triggered by antibodies that induce your body's immune cells to release those histamines again in response to contact with allergens. The most common allergens enter the body through the airway.

If you have allergic rhinitis, you will feel a constant runny nose, ongoing sneezing, swollen nasal passages, excess mucus, weepy eyes, and a scratchy palate and throat. A cough may result from postnasal drip. Some people with allergic rhinitis feel only a drippy nose; others are so congested that the allergy affects every part of their lives. You can often tell a child who has allergic rhinitis by the crease on the top of the nose from constant wiping *(allergic salute)* or dark circles under the eyes *(allergic shiners).*

Infected ears and fluid in the ears because of blocked eustachian tubes are two common results of rhinitis in both adults and children, although the problems are much more common in children. Unending fatigue is another problem and is receiving much attention at this time. Some researchers believe that there is a possible link between allergic rhinitis and chronic fatigue syndrome. Chances are also great that you have achiness, tiredness, and sleep disturbances that result when untreated symptoms interfere with restful sleep.

Seasonal or Perennial

Allergic rhinitis takes two different forms—*seasonal* and *perennial*. When symptoms occur because of trees in the spring, grasses in summer, and weeds in the early fall, they are said to be seasonal. Seasonal allergic rhinitis is usually caused by an allergy to mold spores, grasses, weeds, or pollens from trees and other plants. If you experience year-round rhinitis, you could have perennial allergic rhinitis, or an allergy to environmental dust, dust mites, animal danders, or mold spores or mildew. Your allergic rhinitis can even be triggered by remnants of fur months after a cat, dog, or other pet has been removed from your home.

Overall, seasonal allergic rhinitis is easier to treat because the symptoms are short term; perennial allergic rhinitis from year-round exposure is more difficult to control. If you have both types, you may be prone to recurrent respiratory problems; sinus, throat, and ear infections; tiredness; and irritability.

To diagnose allergic rhinitis, your doctor will do a nasal examination. Your mucous membrane may be swollen, pale, or even whitish-blue in color. The doctor may take a mucus smear to see if it has *eosinophils* (a type of white blood cell characteristic of allergic diseases). Other tests such as those described in Chapter 4 may also be helpful in making the diagnosis.

Common Outdoor Allergens	
Environmental pollution	Pollen
Grass	Ragweed
Industrial pollution	Trees
Mold spores	Weather changes (cold air, fronts, wind, humidity)

Common Indoor Allergens	
Aerosols	Foods
Cosmetics	Fumes
Dander from pets	Mold
Dust	Smoke
Feathers	Wool

Infectious Rhinitis (The Common Cold)

Several hundred different viruses may cause infectious rhinitis, also known as the common cold. These viruses may also affect your airways, sinuses, throat, voice box, and bronchial tubes. A cold usually begins abruptly with great discomfort in your throat followed by such symptoms as clear, watery nasal discharge, sneezing, a tired sensation (malaise), and sometimes fever. Postnasal drip causes the sore throat and cough that accompany colds.

Colds are usually self-limiting and last from three to seven days but occasionally require antibiotics when you also have a bacterial infection. Fatigue, stress, or the virus itself may promote bacterial infection after the body's immune system has been weakened.

Sometimes you may mistake a cold for allergic rhinitis (hay fever) or a sinus infection. If your symptoms begin quickly and are over within one to two weeks, then it is usually a cold, not allergy. If your cold symptoms last longer than two weeks, check with your doctor to see if you have developed an allergy.

Cold or Flu?

How do you know whether it is a cold or flu? Take your temperature. A mild case of the flu often mimics a cold, but a cold rarely raises your temperature above

101 degrees Fahrenheit. Influenza is an acute respiratory infection caused by a variety of influenza viruses and often involves muscle aches and soreness, headache, and fever. Flu viruses enter your body through the mucous membranes of the nose, eyes, or mouth. Every time you touch your hand to one of these areas, you are possibly infecting yourself with a virus; this makes it very important to keep your hands germ-free with frequent washing.

Seeking treatment for colds and flu in the elderly, the very young, or the chronically ill is important. Newer prescription treatments such as rimantadine and amantadine can help to prevent and treat flu infection, although these must be used within forty-eight hours after the start of the illness.

As discussed on page 112, flu vaccines are recommended annually for anyone with respiratory problems, certain chronic illnesses, and particular high-risk groups such as health care providers and those over age sixty-five.

Rhinitis Caused by Medication

Medication rhinitis is due to chemical irritation when you use over-the-counter decongestant nasal sprays for a prolonged period. These sprays relieve nasal congestion by reducing blood flow to the lining of the nose. However, you should only use these for three to five days to avoid worsened swelling of the lining of the nasal passages, destruction of nasal cilia, and changes in the nasal mucus. The symptoms will go away when you stop the drug.

Food Allergy

An estimated 5 percent of the total population has a food allergy. Food allergies in adults are not that common, but children may be more prone to this type of reaction. The most common offenders are cow's milk, corn, eggs, shellfish, peanuts, soybeans, chocolate, celery, wheat products, and chicken. However, food additives used to enhance taste or as preservatives, such as sulfites, nitrites, sodium benzoate nitrates, and monosodium glutamate (MSG), can also cause allergy in sensitive people. BHA/BHT are common preservatives found in cereals or other grain products that cause problems for some allergic people. Tartrazine (FD&C yellow dye no. 5) is another source of problems. This dye is found in many orange or green foods as well as in some medicines colored yellow (see page 23).

If you have a food allergy, you may only feel a mild itchiness in your throat and mouth. Or you may have a more serious and potentially life-threatening reaction called *anaphylaxis*, which may involve swelling of the upper airway with difficulty breathing (see pages 24–26). Some other symptoms you may feel include hives or a rash all over the body, general itchiness, runny nose, asthma, eczema, hives, earaches, drippy eyes, nausea, stomach cramps, vomiting, and diarrhea.

Recent studies show food allergies may contribute to asthma attacks in children. Researchers at Johns Hopkins Children's Center have found that some children with asthma are also highly allergic to one or more foods. Unless the food allergy is controlled, these children may fail to respond to asthma treatment.

An accurate diagnosis of food allergy is important because of the potential for serious, even fatal reactions. If you suspect or know that you are allergic to certain foods, be aware of masked allergens in processed foods, restaurant items, and wines. There have been reported cases of severe anaphylaxis to foods that had trace amounts of offending allergens that were not listed on the package label. Some of these are covered in further detail on pages 161–162.

Tests your doctor may use to detect which foods you are allergic to include total IgE serum level, skin tests, or radioallergosorbent tests (RASTs), which are discussed in Chapter 4.

Common Food Allergens

Alcohol (for example, wine containing sulfites or other allergens)
Berries (usually strawberries, blueberries, raspberries)
Eggs
Fish (usually shellfish, whitefish)
Grains (commonly wheat, gluten, corn, rye)
Milk proteins (can also cause lactose intolerance)
Peanuts
Peppers
Soy
Yeast

Foods Often Containing Tartrazine
(FD&C Yellow Dye No. 5)

Certain breakfast cereals
Cake mixes
Commercial pies
Commercial gingerbread
Chocolate chips
Butterscotch chips
Commercial frostings
Ready-to-eat canned puddings
Certain instant and regular puddings
Certain ice creams and sherbets
Certain candy coatings
Candy drops and hard candies
Colored marshmallows
Flavored carbonated beverages
Flavored drink mixes

Common Foods That May Contain Sulfiting Agents
Restaurant salads (lettuce, tomatoes, carrots, peppers, dressings) Fresh fruit Dried fruits (for example, apricots) Wine, beer, and cordials Alcohol, all sparkling grape juices (including nonalcoholic) Potatoes (for example, French fries, chips) Sausage meats (especially made outside of the United States) Cider and vinegar Pickles Dehydrated vegetables Cheese and cheese mixtures

Anaphylaxis

Anaphylaxis is a very rare but potentially fatal allergic reaction. Symptoms you may feel include:

Flushing
Difficulty breathing
Bronchial spasms
Vomiting
Swelling of the tongue, throat, ear lobes, and nose
Difficulty swallowing
Dangerous drop in blood pressure
Abnormal heart arrhythmias
Hives or welts
Loss of consciousness

If you ever suspect anaphylaxis, it is vital that you seek emergency medical treatment. The symptoms can come on suddenly and dramatically. In severe cases, anaphylaxis can lead to death if not treated in time.

Anaphylaxis is usually treated in the emergency room

with an injection of *epinephrine*. Epinephrine acts quickly to relax the muscles in the bronchi, dilate the airways, improve breathing, stimulate the heart, and reverse hives and swelling in the face. In fact, epinephrine is synonymous with the hormone *adrenaline* produced by the adrenal glands under stress.

There are small, preloaded syringes of epinephrine (EpiPen) available by prescription that you can carry with you in case of a severe reaction to an allergen. Having this convenient syringe can make a life or death difference for someone who has anaphylaxis. If you have a strong history of allergy or have severe reactions to insect bites or certain foods, ask your doctor whether a prescription for this medication would be warranted.

The most common triggers of anaphylaxis are insect stings (bees, ants), foods (shellfish, nuts), or medications. An allergy to latex can sometimes cause an anaphylactic reaction, but it is not as common. You can even suffer anaphylaxis just from breathing the fumes of certain foods. One boy who was severely allergic to corn products experienced dangerous swelling in his throat when friends made microwave popcorn at a birthday party. In another documented case, an eight-year-old girl with multiple food allergies died after inhaling the fumes from a pot of cooking garbanzo beans at a friend's home. Her inhaled bronchodilator medication failed to combat the fatal reaction. Research has documented that inhaling steam from cooking foods can cause breathing problems in susceptible patients who have food allergy.

Peanut allergies are thought to be a leading cause of fatal food reactions, and these usually develop when children are exposed to peanut products during the first years of life. This type of dangerous food allergy may be on the rise because most young children are given peanut butter sandwiches as a quick meal substitute. Unlike allergies to eggs or milk, you do not outgrow the allergy to peanuts and must avoid them for a lifetime.

Exercise-Induced Anaphylaxis

Some people experience an all-over itch and reddened skin that comes on during exercise, called *exercise-induced anaphylaxis*. This potentially fatal condition is an extreme and sudden allergic reaction and can result in death without immediate treatment. Symptoms you may feel with this allergy to exercise include choking, fainting, gastrointestinal problems, itchy skin, and hives.

Many people with exercised-induced anaphylaxis have a strong history of asthma, hay fever, and eczema, and also a family history of allergies. Since exercise-induced anaphylaxis may be life-threatening, you should exercise with someone who understands the problem and treatment, as well as carry a preloaded syringe of epinephrine.

Oral Allergy Syndrome

Some people with allergic rhinitis have oral allergic reactions to fresh fruits and vegetables. This phenomenon has been tagged *oral allergy syndrome* and is suggested to be due to cross-reacting allergens in the foods and pollens. If you are sensitive to the cross-reacting allergens, you may find relief by eliminating certain foods from your diet. Pollens and fruits may share some interesting combinations of cross-reactivity. For example, studies reveal that if you are allergic to avocado, you may also react to bay leaves because they are in the same botanical family. Researchers have found that peas, beans, and licorice allergies may cross-react with peanuts.

If controlling your diet does not provide complete control of symptoms, there are preventive medications available to reduce the reaction. Ask your doctor about sodium cromoglycate that can be administered orally before eating a potentially offending food.

Latex Allergy

Latex allergy is rapidly becoming a growing concern, especially for health care workers such as nurses and lab technicians. According to the American College of Allergy, Asthma, and Immunology, about 18 million Americans, or 64 in every 1,000, are affected by latex sensitivity. This is a dramatic increase from 1 in every 1,000 people in the early eighties. Some recent studies have reported about 17 percent of health care workers being sensitive to latex used in hospital gloves.

This milky sap of the rubber tree *Hevea brasiliensis* is used to make balloons, condoms, diaphragms, elastic for clothing, carpet backing, gloves, and toys. It is also an essential ingredient for many medical and dental tools and devices, including face masks and bandages.

If you have an allergy to latex, you may have experienced skin rashes or minor skin irritation. Some people react more seriously with hives or breathing problems. Rarely, however, does latex allergy produce anaphylactic shock.

Deviated Septum and Nasal Polyps

One source of your breathing problems may be from an anatomical problem such as deviated septum. This occurs when the cartilage and bone in the center of the nose are shifted to one side either from injury or due to a congenital defect. In severe cases, the sinuses are unable to drain on that side of the nose; this leads to a blockage of the sinus channels on that side. Mucus stagnates in the sinus cavity because of the blockage and becomes infected.

Nasal polyps may also be a contributing factor. Polyps develop because of excessive growth of the mucous lining in the nose, especially from one of the turbinates, due to chronic allergic or infectious rhinitis. Nasal polyps can create more barriers to sinus drainage, trap mucus, and create a bacterial breeding ground. They may also affect your sense of smell or taste. What is more important, they may be associated with asthma, especially if you are allergic to aspirin.

A deviated nasal septum may be corrected surgically if the obstruction on one side of your nose is severe. Using a special corticosteroid medicine, which is placed inside the nose by way of a spray, you can shrink nasal polyps. If the medicine does not succeed in shrinking the polyps, they can be removed surgically.

Sinusitis

More than 35 million Americans have sinusitis, or sinus disease. It is a very common chronic disease in the United States and affects more than one out of seven people with more than 16 million visits to doctors' offices annually for treatment. Up to 50 percent of all asthmatics also suffer from chronic sinusitis at some point, which can make asthma symptoms flare and worsen.

Sinus is the medical term for a cavity. The four pairs of sinuses (see page 7), or cavities, in the head (paranasal sinuses) serve an important purpose as they lighten the skull and improve the tonality of your voice. Sinuses must have proper mucus drainage and a functioning immune system to fight off infection. When these are compromised, sinusitis can result.

Sinusitis is an inflammation of the mucous membranes that line the sinus cavities. This inflammation causes the mucous glands in the sinuses to secrete more mucus. When the passages in your sinuses become blocked, pressure develops and your nose may feel plugged. Sinusitis can be caused by a virus, allergic rhinitis (hay fever), chronic rhinitis, deviated nasal septum, or polyps and may run in your family. Irritants, air pollution, smoke, and fumes may also cause inflammation and lead to bacterial growth and infection.

Symptoms of Acute Sinusitis
Headache Pain in the sinus area Upper molar tooth pain Nasal obstruction Postnasal drip Cough Sore throat Thick, yellow or green nasal drainage High fever (102 degrees F and above) Tenderness or dull pain around the eyes and cheek bones

A bacterial infection usually causes acute sinusitis. Chronic sinusitis may not be associated with infection but may be due to other problems as mentioned above. In fact, if you have chronic sinusitis, it may produce a full range of symptoms such as chronic sore throat and cough, particularly when reclining, decreased sense of smell, bad breath, nasal congestion, and a low grade fever (less than 101 degrees Fahrenheit), or it may just produce drainage, sore throat, or a cough that lasts for days to weeks.

The only accurate diagnosis for sinusitis is sinus aspiration and culture. Your doctor will take a sampling of the sinus secretions by one of two methods. A surgeon may use a needle to puncture into a sinus from inside your mouth or nose. Or, a special telescope called an *endoscope* may be used to enter a sinus from inside your nose. By either method, mucus is drawn out and analyzed for causes of infection.

Often the diagnosis depends on your physician's clinical impression. Your physician will do a complete physical examination and take your medical history. Other tests may include taking a special sinus X ray to look for thickening of the membrane lining and clouding because of accumulation of fluid in the sinuses. In some people, sinusitis is associated with asthma, as with sinobronchial syndrome.

Sinobronchial Syndrome

Sinobronchial syndrome is a combination of sinusitis and resultant lower respiratory tract symptoms such as bronchitis or asthma. With this syndrome, the sinus disease can be allergic, acute, or chronic. Likewise, the lung disease can be one of several types such as acute infective bronchitis, recurrent bouts of bronchitis, chronic bronchitis, or asthma that is difficult to control.

It is thought that anywhere from 20 to 70 percent of asthmatic adults also have coexisting sinus disease. Conversely, 15 to 56 percent of those with allergic rhinitis or sinusitis have evidence of asthma. The good news is that researchers have found that treating the sinus disease effectively diminishes the severity and occurrence of the lower airway problems.

The most likely reason for the sinus disease resulting in lower airway symptoms is a constant drip of various inflammatory and infective secretions from the back of the nose to the back of the throat. This throat irritation may cause bronchial constriction by a reflex transmitted by the nervous system. Or, the postnasal drip of inflammatory secretions from the upper airway may create a secondary inflammatory reaction of the lungs, causing either bronchitis or asthma.

If you have sinobronchial syndrome, you will feel a host of miserable symptoms including shortness of breath, wheezing, productive cough, nasal obstruction, fever, headache, or chest tightness. You may have trouble sleeping because lying down causes an increase in the postnasal drainage and an increase in cough. Some people have only mild symptoms such as a cough or chest tightness; others have more severe symptoms, appear quite ill, and are in respiratory distress.

On examination, your doctor may find that you have a rapid respiratory rate, rapid heart rate, and fever. You may have signs of sinus inflammation or infection with tenderness over the sinuses, along with constant nasal and sinus drainage. Your lungs can reveal wheezes or rhonchi, which suggest airway inflammation and the presence of mucus. *Rhonchi* are whistling or snoring sounds heard through the stethoscope when listening to the chest. They indicate a partial obstruction of the airways by mucus or other inflammatory debris such as pus.

Although your chest X ray may show some evidence of airway inflammation, usually most are normal. X rays of your sinuses may reveal chronic inflammatory changes in the sinuses and possibly evidence of infection.

Ask Questions

If you have symptoms of one or more of these common nasal problems, seeing your doctor for an accurate diagnosis is important. Write down any questions and seek answers. Prevention and treatment measures, as outlined throughout this book, can dramatically help to relieve and possibly end the symptoms you experience.

chapter 3

Understanding Asthma and Lung Disorders

Because of scientific breakthroughs in the past few years, we all have a much clearer understanding of what causes the cough, wheezing, shortness of breath, and accompanying inflammation of asthma and other lung diseases. Not only are scientists unraveling these common problems, they have also provided some new medications that go directly to the source and help to control the symptoms without dangerous side effects.

Although we attribute most of the lower airway symptoms to lung disease, sometimes the cause of cough, wheezing, and shortness of breath may be surprising, as Pat, a thirty-eight-year-old mother of three, discovered.

When Pat joined a new dance class at the local community center, she began to have shortness of breath every time she tried to participate. Along with this new symptom, she was frequently awakened at night by cough and wheezing. Pat went from doctor to doctor, searching for relief to these annoying problems, and was prescribed various short-acting inhaled bronchodilators, like albuterol (Ventolin) and oral theophylline (Slo-Bid) for asthma. Yet none of these treatments gave her full relief.

Finally, she went to a respiratory disease specialist who noted that while her spirometry test (page 69) was normal and her airways did not appear obstructed, her chest X ray revealed a small hiatal hernia, which was contributing to heartburn and constant irritation in the throat. A *hiatal hernia* is a protrusion of the stomach up through the diaphragm into the chest. The specialist thought that the short-acting beta2-agonist was not adequate for what seemed to be exercise-induced asthma (EIA). Then, when she went to sleep at night, the theophylline caused problems between the stomach and the esophagus.

After stopping all her past medications, Pat's doctor started her on a new medication regime to stop her symptoms. She began taking salmeterol (Serevent), a long-acting inhaled bronchodilator, every twelve hours. She also took inhaled cromolyn sodium (Intal) about an hour before her dance time. This type of medicine helps to block EIA and has few side effects. Pat took a special antacid pill an hour before bedtime to ease heartburn and end the throat irritation from regurgitated stomach acid. After three months, she dropped the long-acting inhaler and continued to control the stomach acid with medication.

Because of newer means of diagnosing respiratory problems, along with more effective treatments, Pat can now enjoy her dancing without shortness of breath and is sleeping through the night without awakening from gastroesophageal-reflux-induced symptoms (heartburn).

As Pat and millions like her have experienced, there is help once an accurate diagnosis is made. In fact, the outlook for most breathing problems is now remarkably better than even five years ago. New breakthroughs in diagnosing and alleviating these problems are being achieved daily and will improve the prognosis even more for your children and grandchildren.

If you have lung problems, learning all you can about your specific problem is important. Detailed descriptions of the following common lung problems, including risk factors, biological causes, physical symptoms, and diagnosis, will enable you to more fully understand your disease and know when to take appropriate treatment action.

Cough

Cough is one of the most prevalent symptoms of lung disease and stems from many different causes, like postnasal drip, chronic rhinitis, sinusitis, or gastroesophageal reflux (heartburn). With gastroesophageal reflux, the stomach acid regurgitates, or backs up, into the esophagus to cause heartburn, midchest pain, difficulty swallowing, cough, spasm of the larynx, and sometimes asthma. You may have a bitter, burning, or sour stomach taste in your throat or mouth. This is discussed further on pages 52–53.

Asthma is a serious cause of cough that is very common today. Cough-type asthma has been called *hidden asthma* and *cough-variant asthma* and is vastly underdiagnosed and undertreated. Triggers for cough-variant asthma are usually respiratory infections and exercise. You may even have cough-variant asthma and think the cough is due to an allergy. Until an asthma attack occurs, you may not realize how your lungs are involved.

For any persistent cough, even with no other symptoms, contact your doctor. It is helpful to tell your doctor how long the cough has been present, whether any activities or exposures seem to make it worse, whether you notice any other different or unusual feelings, and whether the cough is productive. A cough is *productive* when it brings up phlegm or mucus and *unproductive* when it is dry.

A thorough discussion and physical examination will guide your doctor in ordering tests, such as X ray of your chest; spirometry, which is a pulmonary function test that shows how your lungs are functioning; and blood tests, all of which are explained in Chapter 4. Occasionally, it is necessary to see a pulmonologist (lung specialist) for further tests including *bronchoscopy*, which is a direct examination of your bronchial tubes.

Shortness of Breath

Shortness of breath, or *dyspnea,* is a feeling of breathlessness, or a sense of getting "not enough air," out of proportion to activity. Shortness of breath that is experienced when you are at rest or with little physical activity is not normal and should be brought to the immediate attention of your physician.

There are many causes of shortness of breath. The most common are due to diseases of the lungs or bronchi. Pneumonia, an infection inside the lung itself is associated with the collection of pus (white blood cells) in the alveoli and small bronchial tubes. If this area of diseased lung is large enough, it may cause your feeling of shortness of breath in several ways:

The respiratory muscles must work harder because the lungs are stiffer.

Asthma or bronchitis causes increased airflow resistance so respiratory muscles have more work to do and the expiratory muscles which are normally passive become active to help overcome the airway obstruction.

Nasal passages are blocked.

Because the specific cause of shortness of breath must be

clarified, your doctor will do a physical examination and then order a few tests. These tests may include a chest X ray, tests of lung function, and measurement of oxygen levels in the blood if lung disease is suspected. Other tests may be ordered to evaluate possible heart disease, including an electrocardiogram.

Bronchitis (Acute)

Acute bronchitis is an inflammation and irritation of the bronchial tubes caused by a bacterial or viral infection. You may have a cough with production of sputum, which may be thick and yellow or occasionally blood streaked. You may also have a fever and fatigue, along with wheezing and shortness of breath. If your bronchitis is severe, it may progress into pneumonia, which is inflammation of the lungs due to viral or bacterial infection.

Your doctor will order such diagnostic tests as a chest X ray to make sure no pneumonia is present and blood tests to measure oxygen levels in the blood. Occasionally sputum may be obtained for culture. Your doctor will analyze this under a microscope to find the right treatment such as the choice of antibiotics.

Common Triggers of Bronchitis

Chemical irritants in the air (cigarette smoke, smog, industrial chemicals)
Allergens (triggers that cause allergy)
Infections

Bronchiectasis

Bronchiectasis is abnormal dilation of the bronchial tubes. It is caused by damage to the muscle cartilage and elastic tissue that make up the walls of the medium-sized airways.

Infections such as pneumonia cause this, as do other irritants such as gastroesophageal reflux (heartburn). Bronchiectasis can also occur in cases of cystic fibrosis, which is an inherited disease characterized by a tendency to chronic lung infections and an inability to absorb fats and other nutrients from food. (Cystic fibrosis is discussed in detail on pages 269–71.)

If you have bronchiectasis, you will have a persistent cough because of the accumulation of infected mucus and debris in the distended airways. With bronchiectasis, the cough is productive and the expelled mucus may be discolored and contain blood. You may also experience great fatigue, shortness of breath, and weight loss. Chronic sinusitis is another common symptom that accompanies bronchiectasis.

Understanding the various stages of bronchiectasis is important. Initially, there is injury to the walls of the airways. After this occurs, the immune defenses of the respiratory system weaken. It may be difficult to clear mucus; this makes the airways more susceptible to infection. More infections continue to damage the airway walls and worsen the situation. As with all respiratory diseases, early diagnosis and treatment are important for stopping airway damage.

Your doctor will start by evaluating your medical history and doing a physical exam. Tests that may be helpful in diagnosing bronchiectasis include a chest X ray, pulmonary function tests such as spirometry, and possibly a computerized X ray of the lungs called a CAT scan.

Pneumonia

Pneumonia is inflammation in the lung. There are many different causes of pneumonia; however, infection caused by bacteria or viruses is the most common.

Pneumonia may follow an upper respiratory infection

or flulike illness. You may have a cough, which can be either unproductive (dry) or productive with yellow, green, or bloody phlegm; shortness of breath; fever; and sometimes sharp pains in the chest when you take a deep breath. However, some or all of these signs may not be present. This is especially common in older people or in people who have other underlying medical problems. For example, in elderly adults, fever may not be prominent and the only feeling may be pain in the abdomen.

If there is a persistent cough or fever or if shortness of breath or chest pains occur—especially if these follow another infection—you should contact your doctor. Tests, including chest X ray and sputum examination, can help make the diagnosis. Then, proper treatment of the pneumonia can begin.

The most common cause of pneumonia is a bacteria called Streptococcus pneumoniae or the pneumococcus. Pneumococcal pneumonia can be very serious for those over age sixty-five and for those with problems such as heart disease, lung disease, and diabetes mellitus. Immunization for this type of pneumonia is available and is effective in lowering the risk of this infection (see pages 111–112).

Immunization against the influenza virus is also recommended as discussed on pages 112–113. Yearly influenza immunizations lower the risk for serious influenza infection, especially pneumonia caused by this virus. Pneumonia may also be caused by bacteria, fungi, and other viruses, as well as noninfectious factors.

Chronic Obstructive Pulmonary Disease (COPD)

The term chronic obstructive pulmonary disease (COPD) is commonly used to describe four distinct problems: *asthma, bronchiectasis, chronic bronchitis,* and *emphysema.*

All these conditions have a limitation of airflow and can occur separately or in combination with each other.

The occurrence of chronic bronchitis and emphysema is usually related to cigarette smoking. However, you may develop early emphysema because of an absence of a protective blood component so that chemicals within the body digest the lung at a rapid rate. This may result in symptomatic emphysema in people as early as age thirty and certainly by age fifty.

If you have recurrent respiratory tract infections, exposure to secondhand cigarette smoke or excessive chemical fumes may cause you to develop COPD. Nonetheless, more than 90 percent of those who ultimately develop COPD have acquired it through cigarette smoking. More than 50 percent of lifelong smokers over age fifty show a loss of normal lung function.

There might be some clustering of COPD in families. This would imply that certain persons were at less of a risk of lung damage or COPD with cigarette smoking, whereas others were at higher risk. This possibility aside, the truth remains that the more cigarettes you consume, the higher the risk of lung disease and the more severe the lung disease is if incurred.

Repeated breathing tests have shown that there is loss of lung function as we age. Normally, this occurs at a rate of less than or equal to 1 percent of the lung function per year. So, at age seventy, you would normally have 50 to 60 percent of the breathing capacity that you had at age twenty. In those with COPD, whatever its cause, this deterioration in lung function may occur at a rate of 2 to 3 percent of the lung function per year. This would imply that a 50 percent reduction in lung function may occur by age fifty, resulting in shortness of breath and causing difficulty in exercise and activity.

Common Exacerbations of COPD

An increase or decrease in the sputum produced
An increase in the thickness or stickiness of sputum
A change in sputum color to yellow or green
The presence of blood in the sputum
An increase in the severity of shortness of breath, cough, or wheezing
A general feeling of ill health
Swelling of the ankles
Difficulty sleeping
Using more pillows or sleeping in a chair instead of a bed to avoid
shortness of breath
An unexplained increase or decrease in weight
Increasing morning headaches, dizzy spells, or restlessness
Increased fatigue and lack of energy

Bronchitis (Chronic)

Chronic bronchitis, the sixth leading chronic condition in the United States, usually begins after age thirty-five and affects 13.8 million people. With chronic bronchitis, you have significant sputum or phlegm production on most days. You also experience a cough with sputum (phlegm) for an extended period without another cause such as pneumonia, postnasal drip, or other cause as discussed in this chapter. This is because the chronic, long-term inflammation leaves the airways permanently swollen; this causes them to narrow and produce large amounts of mucus that plugs them up. Because of this inflammation, the mucus glands also enlarge, and this causes profuse secretion of mucus. Moreover, the function of the cilia, which normally helps to clear mucus from the system, is impaired.

The cough associated with chronic bronchitis is worse in the morning after arising. As the disease progresses, your cough may last longer into the day and night. You may also have wheezing and shortness of breath.

Breathing may become increasingly labored as the disease worsens, and the amount of sputum may increase. Some people with COPD have a bluish discoloration of the fingernails because of decreases in the oxygen level in the blood.

Severe bronchitis may result in more serious illnesses such as pneumonia because of bronchial tube obstruction and the inability to cough out infected secretions of mucus. The periods of severe cough and shortness of breath gradually get closer together so that eventually these problems may be continuous. Chronic bronchitis may precede or accompany pulmonary emphysema.

An early diagnosis and proper treatment are important to control chronic bronchitis. Your doctor may order such tests as chest X ray, blood tests to assess your oxygen and carbon dioxide levels, electrocardiogram, and lung function tests. These tests, which are fully explained in Chapter 4, are done to exclude other causes of the problem and to help determine the severity of the chronic bronchitis. Your doctor may also have you cough up a sample of sputum or phlegm and analyze this in a laboratory. This will help determine the infectious cause of the bronchitis and will guide your doctor in prescribing the correct antibiotic.

Treatment measures can bring great relief, keep the disease managed, and allow you to have a good quality of life. These treatments, described in Chapter 5, usually include inhaled beta2-agonists to dilate the bronchial tubes and open the airway, along with inhaled steroids. Sometimes antibiotics are needed for periodic infections, and there are medicines available that help to thin the mucus to make it easier to expel. Sometimes more powerful or more expensive antibiotics are needed. In special cases, your doctor may feel it is necessary to use an oral corticosteroid such as prednisone to reduce the inflammation and resulting mucus production.

Emphysema Due to Cigarette Smoking

Emphysema is an incurable and irreversible disease that is usually caused by cigarette smoke and occurs after age fifty. It affects more than 2.4 million Americans and kills 13,000 people each year in the United States. While more men have emphysema, the disease is increasing in women.

With emphysema, your lung tissues become progressively weakened; this causes air to become entrapped in your lungs (hyperinflation). Although breathing in, or inhaling, is relatively easy with emphysema, you will have trouble breathing out, or exhaling, as your airways constrict or even collapse. These airways may become inflamed and, as with other breathing disorders, get clogged up with mucus.

Over time, emphysema results in a loss of the surface area of the lung, as well as its elasticity, because of destruction of the lung structure around the bronchial tubes. This loss of elasticity causes the air flow out of the lung to be much slower. In turn, the rate at which oxygen can be transferred into the blood stream is reduced.

With emphysema, you may have only a mild cough with clear sputum yet constant difficulty in breathing even with normal activity. Other signs of the disease include fatigue, loss of weight, a barrel-chested look, and overdeveloped neck and shoulder muscles.

Some people with emphysema have chronic bronchitis and asthma, as well; this adds to the obstruction. The control of asthma and treatment of bronchitis are important to keep breathing at an optimum level. New measures can retard or even halt the progress of the disease by preventing further damage and improving the efficiency of the remaining lung tissue.

Stopping cigarette smoking and avoiding pollutants are among the first lines of defense in battling this disease and halting the symptoms. Often, these measures will decrease the subsequent damage to your lungs. Maintaining a regular exercise and activity program is vital to stay in cardiovascular shape. You also need to avoid any further lung infections that could add to the damage. This means treating any respiratory infection early and taking yearly vaccinations for flu, along with Pneumovax, a vaccine to prevent bacteria pneumonia.

Breakthrough methods of treating emphysema are being met with significant optimism. One, in particular, involves surgery to remove part of the lung to reduce the size of the lung (see page 113). The smaller lung fits better inside the chest and helps to make breathing easier by allowing the respiratory muscles to work more efficiently.

Emphysema: Inherited

Alpha-1 antitrypsin (A1AT) deficiency is a genetic, or hereditary, condition in which a shortage of a certain protein in the bloodstream may predispose you to several illnesses, including emphysema (or a breakdown of the lung tissue), chronic liver problems, or more rarely, a skin condition called panniculitis (in which inflammatory ulcers develop in the fat underneath the skin). Severe deficiency of this protein is responsible for approximately 3 percent of all cases of emphysema and is surprisingly common; there are estimates that 80,000 to 100,000 Americans are affected. Yet, alpha-1 antitrypsin deficiency is frequently underrecognized. Surveys suggest that those with alpha-1 antitrypsin deficiency may experience symptoms for an average of seven years and see many doctors before the diagnosis is made.

Of the three illnesses associated with alpha-1 antitrypsin deficiency—emphysema, chronic liver disease, and panniculitis—the most common is emphysema, and so alpha-1 antitrypsin deficiency is sometimes called genetic emphysema.

The main symptom of emphysema is shortness of

breath. Other symptoms include cough, phlegm or mucus production, wheezing, and swelling of the feet, which may accompany strain placed on the heart when the oxygen in the bloodstream is low.

Cigarette smoking dramatically accelerates the onset of shortness of breath and emphysema in those with alpha-1 antitrypsin deficiency, so avoidance of cigarette smoking is very important. Fortunately, despite having blood levels below the protective threshold level, not everyone with severe A1AT deficiency develops emphysema, especially if he or she has never smoked.

Breathing tests, such as spirometry, are very important in diagnosing and evaluating both types of emphysema. The chest X ray can also reveal signs of emphysema by showing a loss of visible blood vessels and lung tissue (so-called hyperlucency of the lung). If you have emphysema *not* caused by A1AT deficiency, these changes are most commonly evident at the *upper portions* of the lungs. However, if you have emphysema due to A1AT deficiency, the changes are more evident at the *bottoms,* or *bases,* of the lungs. A suspicion of A1AT deficiency can be confirmed by a simple blood test.

Clues That Indicate Suspicion of Alpha-1 Antitrypsin Deficiency

Emphysema occurring at an early age (less than forty-five years)

Emphysema with chest-X-ray changes at the bottom or bases of the lungs

Emphysema that occurs in a nonsmoker or in an individual who has smoked very little

A family history of emphysema, especially in a non- or minimal smoker

A history of emphysema and liver disease that occurs either in the same individual or within the same family

A history of liver disease that is not explained by other common causes (for example, hepatitis infection and excessive alcohol use)

A history of panniculitis (inflammatory ulcers of the skin)

Asthma

Asthma is a Greek word initially used by Hippocrates nearly 2,200 years ago to describe episodes of shortness of breath. Although the treatments have vastly changed since then, the disease is still the same—a chronic inflammatory disease of the airways.

If you have asthma, you know how frightening the symptoms of wheezing, coughing, shortness of breath, and chest tightness can be. However, breakthrough advances in our understanding of asthma have shifted the emphasis of treatment from just controlling the symptoms to an early use of medications to control airway inflammation.

A serious global health problem, asthma affects nearly 100 million people worldwide. This intermittent, reversible illness is the seventh-ranking chronic condition in the United States. Annually, the disease accounts for 15 million physician visits, 479,000 hospitalizations, 1.2 million emergency room visits, and 10 million missed days at school.

The negative impact of asthma on your physical, social, and emotional life can be considerable. Inadequate asthma management can limit your ability to exercise and participate in sports that demand stamina and physical fitness. You may experience fatigue due to frequent asthma-related sleep disturbances. Furthermore, if your asthma is poorly controlled, it can lead to multiple visits to the emergency room, and also hospital admission that may adversely affect your performance at work or at home.

Rise in Mortality

Even though there are seemingly miraculous treatments for the symptoms of asthma, it is a dangerous disease. Most recently, asthma deaths have dramatically increased despite the newer methods of diagnosis and treatment. The latest estimates from the Centers for Disease Control and Prevention (CDC) reveal that the overall age-adjusted death rate for asthma in 1991 was 18.8 per 1 million population (5,106 deaths), which was 40 percent higher than the similar estimate in 1982 (13.4 per million, or 3,154 deaths).

The rise in asthma mortality has disproportionately affected the poor and minority ethnic groups. This is thought to be because many children with asthma in this population have never seen a doctor, received the proper diagnosis, or had proper medications to treat the airway constriction and inflammation.

In many cases, significant sources of allergens such as cockroaches, dust mites, animals, and rodents are not controlled in these populations; this adds to the increasing rise in the incidence of disease and mortality.

Mechanisms of Asthma

In asthma, your airways are "twitchy" and become inflamed when they meet such stimuli as allergens or cold air. When you have an attack, spasms of the bronchial muscles, along with swelling of the mucousal membrane lining the bronchi and excessive amounts of mucus, contribute to airway narrowing. Consequently, the airway resistance and the work of breathing increases to cause wheezing and shortness of breath. You may have a cough due to irritation inside the airway and the body's attempt to clean out the accumulations of mucus.

Why you have airway inflammation and bronchial hyperreactivity and others do not is unclear. Allergy clearly plays an important role in many asthma cases but not in all. As with allergy, you can blame your family history; there is a strong genetic tie for asthma.

Classification of Asthma

Asthma is primarily classified as either *extrinsic* or *intrinsic*. *Extrinsic asthma* develops early if you have a personal and family history of allergy. Other distinguishing features are increased numbers of certain white blood cells called *eosinophils,* elevated levels of IgE antibodies, and predictable seasonal variation in symptoms. Generally, the severity of extrinsic asthma lessens as you grow older.

Intrinsic asthma, in contrast, usually begins in adulthood, exhibits little or no seasonal variation, and is not associated with allergies. A family history of asthma is also less important. Intrinsic asthma tends to worsen with age, and some people who have had the disease for long periods of time develop irreversible airway obstruction.

Asthma Triggers

Triggers are the factors that cause your asthma attack by initiating airway inflammation and bronchospasm. Your asthma triggers will not be the same as someone else's and can even vary at different times in your life. However, it is important to know your specific asthma triggers to manage this disease effectively.

Signs and Symptoms

Although many people have the onset of asthma in early childhood, first asthma symptoms can occur at any age. Typically, you will experience episodes of cough and shortness of breath with intervals of complete remission. A nonproductive cough and wheeze often accompany the onset of asthma attack. After a period of time, you may suddenly experience the sensation of suffocation and chest tightness. Some people with asthma only experience a cough.

Asthma Triggers: Factors That Exacerbate Asthma		
ASTHMA TRIGGER	EXAMPLES	COMMENTS
1. Respiratory infections	Viral Bacterial Chlamydial	Are a very common cause of exacerbation especially in children under age ten. Bronchial hyperresponsiveness can last as long as two months after an upper respiratory infection.
2. Allergens	Domestic mites Cockroaches Animals (cat, dog) Pollens Fungal spores	Asthma exacerbation after dust exposure is usually due to mite allergy. Plant derived pollens are a common cause of hay fever and contrary to popular belief only occasionally cause asthma exacerbation. Airborn fungal spores may be more important allergens than pollens.
3. Environmental factors	Pollution Sulfur dioxide Nitrogen oxide Ozone Cold temperature High humidity	Asthma symptoms and hospital admissions are increased during periods of heavy air pollution.
4. Physical activity	Vigorous exercise	Bronchoconstriction peaks five to ten minutes after the cessation of exercise and lasts for up to sixty minutes.
5. Drugs and food additives	Aspirin NSAID Beta blockers Tartrazine Metabisulfite Monosodium glutamate (MSG)	Aspirin allergy is commonly associated with nasal polyps. Beta blockers used to treat high blood pressure can trigger an asthma attack. Food additives are a rare cause of asthma exacerbation.

Asthma Triggers: Factors That Exacerbate Asthma (cont.)		
ASTHMA TRIGGER	EXAMPLES	COMMENTS
6. Emotional factors	Stress	Although stress can trigger an asthma attack, it is not a psychosomatic disease: if you don't have asthma, stress cannot make you have it.
7. Others	Smoking Perfumes Sprays Paints Alcohol Pregnancy Menses	Secondhand smoking is an important cause of asthma exacerbation. Children with asthma exposed to maternal smoking need more asthma medications and more frequently visit emergency rooms with acute symptoms. Some alcohol-containing beverages contain metabisulfite that may cause asthma. Occasionally alcohol by itself induces bronchospasm.

The severity of asthma attacks and symptoms varies from time to time and person to person. If you have had asthma for a long time, you may experience chronic cough, wheezing, and decreased stamina during exercise. You may even develop asthma symptoms when you are laughing or singing. Many have a worsening of airflow obstruction at night and in the early morning hours for reasons that are still unclear (see Chapter 9 on sleep-related asthma).

If you look back to a time when you had an asthma attack, usually you will find an exposure to some trigger before the onset of symptoms. Although the onset of a cough, shortness of breath, or wheezing is gradual in most people, in a few people, life-threatening airflow obstruction may develop within a matter of a few hours. This is especially true for about 15 percent of those with asthma who are not aware of the degree of the severity of their airway obstruction. Frequently, these people rush to the emergency room with severe airflow obstruction. They may have a higher risk for asthma-related complications, such as a need for mechanical ventilation, air leaks from the lung (pneumothorax), and even death.

Some types of asthma are potentially fatal, such as *status asthmaticus*. This is associated with dangerous mucus accumulation or plugging in smaller bronchi. It is important to be aware of this type asthma and prevent it with early intervention that deals with the inflammatory component of asthma. Status asthmaticus does not respond quickly to routine treatment (inhaled bronchodilators, injected epinephrine, or intravenous theophylline). Corticosteroid therapy may need to be prolonged with this severe form.

Have you ever suffered an asthma attack and then by the time you got to the doctor's office or emergency clinic, the cough, wheeze, and shortness of breath were gone? You've got a lot of company! Surprisingly, asthma is very difficult to diagnose during a physical examination. Wheezing and hyperinflation of the chest usually happen during an asthma attack. But these symptoms may be gone by the time your doctor listens to your chest. Nasal polyps may be a clue to asthma if you have aspirin-induced bronchospasm.

Wheezing is considered a nonspecific finding; therefore, a careful examination to exclude other diseases that may cause shortness of breath and wheezing is usually done in everyone with suspected asthma. Although you might show a "normal" chest X ray, that does not mean asthma is excluded. While your airflow may be "normal" at your doctor's office, this one-time measurement does not reflect the severity of airflow obstruction during an attack. In fact, there is evidence that some people are more accurate in estimating the severity of airflow limitation than their physicians. The best way to measure how well you can breathe is to perform spirometry or peak flow metering (see pages 69–73).

Asthma Mimics

While cough, wheezing, and shortness of breath are nonspecific symptoms of bronchial asthma, a variety of diseases can also cause them. Two of these conditions warrant special attention.

Cardiac Asthma

Cardiac asthma is commonly mistaken for bronchial asthma. It is a form of heart failure in which the part of the heart muscle that receives blood from the lungs is weakened. Recurrent wheezing and difficulty breathing result from this passive congestion of the lungs and bronchial mucous membranes, which causes narrowing of airways. The symptoms of cardiac asthma usually show up at night after a few hours sleep when blood has been redistributed from the legs and lower body back to the lungs and heart. They are relieved a few minutes after you assume an upright position. If you have cardiac asthma, you may show mild bronchial hyperreactivity after inhaling a drug called *methacholine*. Occasionally, you may experience some improvement in symptoms after bronchodilator inhalation. However, improvement after using a bronchodilator is not as great in cardiac asthma as in bronchial asthma.

The possibility of cardiac asthma should be considered

in all adults with new-onset asthma. Careful physical examination may reveal findings suggesting heart failure. Chest X ray, electrocardiogram, and evaluation of cardiac function may be undertaken whenever diagnosis is in doubt.

Vocal Cord Dysfunction

Many recent reports have drawn attention to a peculiar syndrome in which a dysfunction of the vocal cords causes wheezing that is frequently misdiagnosed as asthma. This syndrome is most common in young females who have loud and dramatic episodes of wheezing that do not respond to bronchodilators. Some experts believe it to be a manifestation of some type of psychiatric problem.

Warning Signs and Symptoms of Asthma or Status Asthmaticus

Increased frequency of wheezing and dyspnea
Decreasing ability to exercise
Cough productive of sputum that is getting thicker
Shortness of breath
Restlessness
Wheeze or cough, especially at night or after exercise
Feeling of tightness in the chest
Worsened sleep quality because of wheezing or attacks of breathlessness
More frequent use of bronchodilator drugs
Fast breathing (hyperventilation)

Gastroesophageal Reflux Disease (GERD) and Asthma

Recent studies show that up to 89 percent of those with asthma also suffer from heartburn or gastroesophageal reflux disease. GERD generally occurs at night when the sufferer is lying down. Normally a valve between the esophagus and the gastric system prevents stomach acids from backing up into the esophagus. In GERD, the valve does not function properly. The stomach acids reflux, or back up, into the esophagus; this causes irritation and inflammation that can trigger an asthma attack. Sometimes, if the acidic liquids are aspirated, the lungs can also become inflamed and develop a certain type of pneumonia.

Certain clues that suggest reflux as the cause of asthma include the onset of asthma in adulthood, no family history of asthma, no history of allergies or bronchitis, difficult-to-control asthma, or coughing while lying down. Interestingly, the theophylline-containing bronchodilators may even worsen GERD because they relax the valve between the stomach and esophagus. With GERD, an individual may experience the typical reflux symptoms of heartburn, regurgitation, indigestion, and belching. Uncommon symptoms include chest pain, sore throat, hoarseness, and laryngitis. Children may exhibit such symptoms as nocturnal coughing or wheezing, pain in the pit of the stomach, or wheezing after vomiting as signs of reflux-induced asthma.

Tests used to diagnose GERD include a medical examination and personal history. Your doctor may request an esophageal manometry. This test involves measuring the pressures inside the esophagus and stomach. A twenty-four-hour esophageal pH test may also be useful as it verifies whether stomach acid refluxes to the esophagus. At times, a special type X ray may be necessary to see the esophagus and how it functions during swallowing.

Your doctor will probably encourage you to record asthma and reflux symptoms, along with your peak expiratory flow rates. Treatment can include medication to stop the overproduction of stomach acid. In some cases, surgery may be necessary to correct the problem.

Exercise-Induced Asthma

Exercise-induced asthma (EIA) or exercise-induced bron-chospasm (EIB) is also common, occurring in up to 90 percent of all persons with asthma. If you have EIA, you will feel chest tightness, coughing, and difficulty breathing within the first five to eight minutes of an aerobic work-out. These symptoms usually subside in the next twenty to thirty minutes of exercise, but up to 50 percent of those with EIA may have another asthma attack six to ten hours later.

Remember how the nose is important for warming air as it enters the airways? With exercise, most people take in very rapid, shallow breaths through the mouth instead of the nose. This forces cold, dry air down into the bronchial tubes. A reaction then takes place in which the mast cells in the bronchial mucosal linings become unstable and release inflammatory agents or mediators such as hista-mine. Once this reaction occurs, it causes the smooth muscles to contract; this results in shortness of breath, wheezing, and cough.

Everyone needs regular exercise. If you have an allergy or asthma, exercise helps to keep your body conditioned and strong. Yet it is important always to premedicate before exercise and activity to keep symptoms from hap-pening. Many have had great success with some newer inhaled medications, as discussed in Chapter 5.

Occupational Asthma

Occupational asthma results from triggers associated with your work environment. Commonly, you may have asth-matic attacks Monday through Friday but not Saturday and Sunday when you are home from work.

If you have occupational asthma, you may not have the classic asthma symptoms of wheezing and shortness of breath. Many people have rhinitis or eye irritation or develop a cough rather than wheezing. Others complain of unending tiredness, and some have a delayed allergic reaction to something at work, yet do not develop symptoms until they are home. Conversely, with occupational asthma, your symptoms will often subside after a week or more away from the workplace. For those who do not take long vacations, they may never enjoy a disease-free period.

Common Vocations Associated with Occupational Asthma

Animal breeders	Laxative manufacturers
Bakers	Manufacturers
Detergent manufacturers	Metal workers, metal platers,
Dye workers	welders
Epoxy resin, paint, chemical	Nurses, hospital workers
workers	Painters, foam manufacturers
Farmers	Pharmaceutical workers
Food processors	Plastic workers
Food wrappers	Printers
Grain handlers	Textile workers
Hairdressers	Woodworkers, carpenters
Laboratory workers	

Reactive Airways Dysfunction Syndrome (RADS)

When occupational asthma happens after a usually brief and traumatic exposure to high concentrations of irritant fumes, gases, or chemicals, it is called *reactive airways dysfunction syndrome*.

RADS is identical to asthma but is triggered by exposure to chemicals. This commonly occurs when laboratory workers are exposed to chemicals and react with asthma-like symptoms, or when fire fighters start wheezing after being overcome by smoke inhalation.

Your physician can begin to diagnose occupational asthma by first taking your personal history. Overall, a physical examination is not particularly useful because asthma is an illness that tends to wax and wane. You may be without signs such as wheezing, shortness of breath, or cough at the time you see your doctor and then start wheezing Monday morning when you are back on the job. In cases such as these, a tentative diagnosis might be made, and your positive response to asthma medications would support this diagnosis.

Your doctor may have you measure your lung function before and after a work shift, using a peak flow meter (see pages 70–73). However, sometimes the asthma response is delayed by several hours and can be missed. Therefore, measuring PEFR (peak expiratory flow rate) over a period of time, including times away from work, is necessary to detect the decline in lung function.

Until recently, it was widely believed that asthma was a condition of *reversible airway obstruction*. However, it is now clear that the inflammation that accompanies the obstruction can lead to a permanent deterioration in lung function. It is very important to identify asthma of any cause and treat it aggressively. This means avoiding any known triggers that cause the asthma symptoms. Frequently with occupational asthma, removing yourself from exposure is adequate treatment. Sadly, by the time many people with occupational asthma see their physicians, the airway disease is often irreversible and even removal from the work-related trigger does not cure the disease. This gives even greater reason to have your respiratory problem diagnosed early and effective treatment begun when it is most likely to work.

Solving the Mystery of Asthma

It is exciting to see the groundbreaking research as scientists unravel the mystery of lung diseases. Some new studies on asthma have revealed that a gene that causes the lungs to become inflamed and constricted is on the same region of a chromosome where researchers previously found another frequent contributor to asthma—a gene that controls levels of IgE that is associated with allergic reactions. This discovery from Johns Hopkins University gives new insight into the genetic causes of asthma and may help give new clues for treatment.

According to a study from the Dean Foundation for Health, Research, and Education in Madison, Wisconsin, adults who develop asthma may be infected with a type of bacteria that could be treated with antibiotics. Although adults who develop asthma often don't have underlying allergies, this study is being given further attention to see whether adult asthma may be caused by an allergic reaction to the bacteria chlamydia pneumoniae, which can cause sore throat, bronchitis, and pneumonia.

No matter what lung problem you have, it is important to seek an accurate diagnosis from a health care professional who understands the disease. As you will read in the next section, there are some proven, positive steps you can take to get back in control and find excellent relief for most breathing problems.

Part 2

Getting Back in
Control

chapter 4

Taking Responsibility for Self-Care

"I quit!" That is what twenty-one-year-old Kim told her college softball coach after having an asthma attack during a recent playoff game. As had happened many times before, Kim's over-the-counter inhaler wore off as she was running the bases to score for her team. Instead of touching home plate in victory, Kim collapsed midstride, panicked because she could not catch her breath.

Who blames Kim for wanting to quit? It's easy to feel like giving up when you battle breathing problems day after day, year after year, isn't it? Especially after a bout with a cold, it seems as if the chest tightness, shortness of breath, and constant congestion will never end. Just when you feel like it is improving, a viral infection attacks your respiratory system with vengeance and produces more congestion, wheezing, and cough. However, *getting back in control* is important to better breathing, and everyone deserves that!

"How can I be a college athlete when my allergies and asthma control me?" Kim asked her doctor. "The slightest trigger sets off a deluge of mucus pouring out of my sinuses and coughing and wheezing that take my breath away." Through an asthma education program provided by her doctor, Kim learned that control *is* possible. But to gain control, she had to take the first step by accepting personal responsibility for her illness.

Some people hesitate to seek help for breathing problems as they feel their condition cannot be treated easily. In Kim's case, she was unaware of the new prescription medications that can prevent episodes of shortness of breath altogether and depended instead on unreliable over-the-counter preparations. Still, some people simply deny that there is a problem until it becomes serious. Richard was one such man.

Richard, a sixty-four-year-old attorney and cigarette smoker for forty years, has a strong history of COPD in his family. Not only did his father have chronic bronchitis and emphysema, but Richard's two brothers and an uncle, also smokers, got this disease later in life, too.

Several years ago, Richard began to have shortness of breath and cough when he walked from his car to his office building. Not wanting to admit he had a family tendency toward lung disease, he attributed this to being overweight and vowed to watch his diet. On the golf course, Richard would always be behind his friends, dragging his golf cart. When his buddies would ask why he was out of breath all the time, Richard would laugh it off, saying, "Because my body is crying out for another cigarette."

Yet at Richard's sixtieth birthday party, he found out how short of breath he was, and this time he was not laughing. As he went to blow out the sixty candles on his birthday cake, Richard realized he could not get much air out of his lungs. In fact, he could only get enough breath to blow the candles out one at a time.

As the candles were slowly extinguished, the severity of his breathing problem became apparent to family and friends. By the time the last candle was put out, Richard felt lightheaded and dizzy and could not catch his breath.

The next day Richard saw his family doctor who asked about his family history and did a physical examination. The doctor ordered a series of tests, including a chest X ray, a pulmonary function test, and blood tests to check his oxygen levels. A few days later, the tests all confirmed what Richard already knew: chronic obstructive pulmonary disease.

Do not think this is a depressing story! Today, at age sixty-four, Richard does *not* struggle to breathe and he does *not* fear his disease. In fact, he says he feels like a new man and works out with weights and on a stationary bicycle at a nearby health club several times a week. Richard quit smoking cigarettes cold turkey on his sixtieth birthday; this greatly decreased his symptoms. Since his diagnosis, he successfully uses a combination of inhaled medications, including ipratropium (Atrovent) and albuterol (Ventolin), along with triamcinolone (Azmacort), an inhaled steroid spray. All these help to open his airways and ease his shortness of breath.

Richard now sees his doctor regularly, checks his peak flow rate daily, and gets an annual influenza vaccine. When Richard had a tough time with bronchitis last winter, he was able to "weather the storm," as he put it, by taking oral steroids for a short period of time to reduce the swelling and open the airways.

Richard finally took responsibility for his health. With his doctor's help, he is in control of his disease, and his quality of life has soared! If you have a respiratory problem, control starts when you actively seek an accurate diagnosis, regularly take the prescribed medications your doctor gives you, become aware of any abnormal symptoms and report these to your doctor, avoid triggers with environmental control, exercise regularly, eat healing foods, and get restful, healing sleep, among others.

Quite honestly, *no one* can help you breathe right if you don't take the *first step*. And self-efficacy, or having a feeling of controlling your life (and your breathing!), is essential to good health and a higher quality of life.

Working with Your Doctor

Your doctor plays the first most significant role as you get in control of your problem. Not only does he or she serve as the one who can accurately diagnose and prescribe treatment for your problem, this health care professional may become a close, dependable friend to talk to when concerns turn into ongoing worries and anxieties. Because of the widespread growth of managed care, finding the right person to diagnose and treat breathing disorders properly and cost-effectively is not always easy. The following suggestions may offer insight.

Primary Care Physician

Carefully choose a physician whom you can trust to know your medical history very well and take responsibility for your overall health care. This general practitioner, pediatrician, or internist is your primary doctor and is better able to assess your problems and make the necessary referrals to a specialist—an allergist; ear, nose, and throat specialist; or pulmonologist (lung doctor)—if you need further treatment or special care.

After selecting a primary care physician, many people question whether they also need a specialist. As a rule, if your response to treatment is unsatisfactory and the lack of good control of symptoms still interferes with your quality of life, you may consider talking with a specialist. Especially when coexisting illnesses or treatment complicate the management of your problem and you are experiencing loss of days from school or work, you should consult a specialist.

Be aware that problems may occur when you have more than one doctor administering treatment. Unless effective communication takes place between the physicians, you may find yourself in a precarious situation as far as your health is concerned. For example, your allergist may prescribe a certain antihistamine to help control your runny nose. Yet when you develop an upper respiratory infection, your primary physician, or family doctor, may write a prescription for the antibiotic erythromycin. This combination of medications is potentially dangerous and can cause irregular heart rhythms and other serious problems. While both doctors are working at making you well, it is important to have one doctor who knows all about you—your condition, your symptoms, your treatment plan, and the specific medications you are taking. It must be emphasized that a knowledgeable patient who reports the details, including changes in medications, to each doctor will help her- or himself.

Specialists Who Treat Respiratory Problems

PRIMARY CARE PHYSICIAN A general practitioner, family practice doctor, pediatrician, or internist who has completed three years of training after medical school graduation

ALLERGIST A pediatrician or internist who has taken additional training to qualify as a specialist in allergy and immunology after completing training as an internist

INTERNIST A doctor who specializes in internal medicine, the study of diseases in adults, particularly those related to internal organs, and who has completed three years of training after medical school

OTOLARYNGOLOGIST An ear, nose, and throat specialist who treats problems with those and related structures of the head and neck and who has trained four to five years in this field after medical school

PEDIATRICIAN A physician who has three years of special training in the field of pediatrics after medical school graduation

---

Specialists Who Treat Respiratory Problems (cont.)

PULMONARY REHABILITATION THERAPIST A nurse or respiratory therapist who is trained in pulmonary rehabilitation techniques, such as patient education, exercise, pulmonary physiotherapy, stress reduction, and support

PULMONOLOGIST An internist who has taken two or three additional years of training to qualify as a specialist in respiratory diseases and critical care medicine

---

Age, Sex, and Credentials

In choosing a health care professional, some people ask friends for recommendations, check the physician's credentials, or call the local hospital for referrals. In this age of managed care, you will need to check the list of doctors who will accept your insurance provider. Nevertheless, none of these methods is foolproof for finding a qualified professional with whom you can feel comfortable to share your innermost feelings and concerns about your health problems.

Perhaps one of the most important steps to take when selecting this health care professional is to know yourself, including your personal likes and dislikes. Do you feel more comfortable with a man or woman? Should your physician be older than you, the same age, or younger? Do you have a preference as to educational background? These questions are important to consider when making your appointment.

Ask the following questions as you go through the process of choosing a physician.

Is the doctor board certified (passed a standard exam given by the governing board in his or her specialty)?

Where did the doctor go to medical school? (Your local medical society can provide this information.)

Is the doctor involved in any academic pursuits, such as teaching, writing, or research? (This doctor may be more up-to-date in the latest developments in his field.)

At which hospitals does the doctor have hospital privileges, and where are these hospitals located? (Some doctors may not be able to admit patients to certain hospitals, and this is an important consideration for those with chronic health problems.)

Does the doctor accept your type health insurance, or is the doctor a member of the medical panel associated with your HMO?

The Consultation

Plan an initial consultation with the doctor during which you can get to know each other. This will include a detailed interview and physical examination. Patient-physician communication is important to receive the highest quality of care, and also comfort needed during anxious moments.

During this initial interview ask questions as to the preferred methods of treatment. Does the physician appear to relate well to people? Do you feel at ease in talking with the doctor? Are your questions answered? Is she or he current in using the latest methods of treatment?

Especially with a chronic illness, your physician needs to be accessible. When you are ill, popularity is not important but availability is. Make sure your choice of a physician yields a person who is not only an excellent doctor but also available and attentive to your personal needs. Does the doctor allow ample time with you so that quality care is received? Are your questions answered clearly, and are necessary tests made?

Check on office hours, and make sure these fit with your daily schedule. How is payment made? What insurance providers are accepted? Ask for information about emergency availability and charges. Is your doctor always on call or are other doctors sharing coverage? Even the receptionist's responses may set the tone and help you decide if this is the right office. The support staff will be the ones who help you most with prescriptions, obtaining necessary lab work and X rays, and making appointments with hospitals or other professional services.

And let's not forget to mention that doctors are not perfect. Medical errors can result in undertesting, when the doctor does not ask for enough tests to make an accurate evaluation. Great expense can be incurred, when the doctor requests far more tests than necessary. Clearly, there is only one way to make sure you receive excellent care and that is to be assertive and knowledgeable as you take responsibility for your health.

Changes in medical coverage may mean that the doctor you see now will not be the one you see in a year or two. This makes it even more important to understand your particular problem fully, stay abreast of treatment methods, and fully follow the management plan as discussed in this book.

Specialized Tests

Once you have selected the physician to treat your illness, she or he will seek an accurate diagnosis by obtaining a detailed medical history. This will include information on symptoms, how you feel, known asthma and allergy triggers, your activity level and diet, your home and work environment, and family history, and then doing a thorough medical examination.

During this evaluation, it is important that you talk openly with your doctor to interpret the results of the interview and the physical examination, laboratory testing, and X rays. This will allow you to have a firm understanding of your breathing problems and will be the basis for your knowledge of the suggested plan of treatment.

Trust your doctor to decide which set of tests is best in your case to ensure no other medical problems are present. This can help you avoid extra testing that may add little to your diagnosis and only increases the number of tests and expense. If you fear one specific diagnosis, such as lung cancer, be sure you tell your doctor. If you still do not feel comfortable with the diagnosis, talk to your doctor and then have more testing. Or, get a second opinion until you have peace of mind that the problem has been diagnosed correctly. Then, proper treatment can begin.

Getting back in control of your illness depends on an accurate diagnosis. Once the disease is properly identified, your doctor can prescribe a treatment regime that can *prevent and relieve your problems.*

The following tests are commonly used to assess the degree of impairment and monitor the effectiveness of treatment.

Spirometry

Spirometry, which measures how much air you can exhale, is the most accurate pulmonary function test used in confirming the presence of reversible airway obstruction. It can accurately measure the degree of impairment of a person's lung function. When using the spirometer, you will be asked to breathe in and out of a hose attached to a mouthpiece. A small computer measures this amount of air on newer spirometers. The standard measurement is the *FEV-1,* or forced expiratory volume in one second. This is the amount of air exhaled in one second after taking a breath. This test can also monitor your response to medications and is recommended for adults and children over age five.

Peak Flow Testing

Although spirometry is the standard method for the objective evaluation of lung function in the office setting, most experts recommend regular home peak expiratory flow rate (PEFR) measurement for self-assessment of asthma control by patients because it provides a reliable objective measure of bronchial tube function.

PEFR is the highest airflow velocity that you can achieve during a forced expiration starting from maximum inspiration. PEFR is expressed in liters per minute; the normal range for men is from 500 to 700 liters per minute and for women, from 380 to 500 liters per minute. PEFR is effort dependent and is affected by age, sex, race, and smoking.

When done accurately, a drop in the peak flow measurement reflects an obstruction in the large airways. For example, if you were a woman and your normal peak flow measurement was 500, a drop to 375 would show worsening of your illness. Using the scale given on page 71, you would be in the yellow zone and would need to increase your asthma treatment. If the measurement dropped even further to 250, you would be in the red zone and should call your doctor immediately for instructions.

The PEFR is less accurate than office spirometry. But for serial monitoring of lung function, this convenient peak flow monitoring is acceptable and can help you manage your symptoms at home.

A variety of small and inexpensive devices are available for home PEFR monitoring and not only are essential for asthma but may be useful for the management of chronic bronchitis and emphysema. This instrument, called a *peak flow meter* (see page 73), is a small tube with a mouthpiece on one end, a place for air to escape on the other end, and a calibrated meter on the side. When you blow air from your lungs into the tube, a small marker moves along the meter or scale and stops at a certain point. This point indicates your peak expiratory flow rate (PEFR) and provides an objective assessment of how well you are breathing. This rate will let you know whether you need more medication or your asthma symptoms are under control.

Most devices function satisfactorily for up to one or two years. The device should be regularly cleaned with soap and warm water according to the manufacturer's specifications

---

Color-Coded PEFR Zones

GREEN ZONE: ABSENCE OF SYMPTOMS

If your PEFR is in the green zone, you should have no symptoms. This means that your PEFR is between 80 to 100 percent of your personal best, and there is no need to make any treatment change. After a sufficient period of stability, you might attempt to cut back on asthma medications.

YELLOW ZONE: CAUTION

If your PEFR is in the yellow zone, PEFR of 50 to 80 percent of your personal best, this means your asthma is worsening. You need to temporarily increase the treatment.

RED ZONE: WARNING

If your PEFR is in the red zone, PEFR less than 50 percent of your personal best, this shows that your symptoms are worsening enough to require immediate bronchodilator administration. Call your doctor. You may need a rescue course of oral steroids. Try to look for exposure to some unsuspected allergen(s) and carefully review the medications you are taking with your doctor.

Peak Expiratory Flow Rate Monitoring in Asthma

WHO NEEDS PEFR MONITORING

Anyone older than five who has moderate to severe asthma. Especially useful for those who cannot tell when the symptoms such as cough or tightness in chest are starting.

WHICH DEVICE TO USE

Any commercially available device. Usual cost ranges from $15 to $25. Use the same brand for all future use. Electronic PEFR devices are considerably more expensive and do not offer any major advantage over handheld devices.

HOW TO MEASURE PEFR

Carefully follow the recommended procedure:
Stand up or sit in an upright position.
Take a deep breath to inflate the lungs fully.
Place the end of PEFR monitor in the mouth.
Tightly close the lips around the mouth piece.
Blow out as fast and as hard as possible.
Write down the value of PEFR.
Repeat the same maneuver three times.
Record the highest of the three values.

HOW TO GET STARTED

Measure the PEFR at least twice per day, in the morning and evening.
Measure PEFR consistently either before or after the bronchodilator use.
Establish your personal best value.
After you establish asthma control, reduce the frequency of PEFR monitoring to once a day, preferably early in the morning after waking up.

The PEFR maneuver is easy to learn. With minimum training, most patients older than five can master the technique and keep an accurate record. The important aspects of PEFR monitoring with asthma are summarized on page 70. A sample chart is shown on page 74. In both normal people and those with asthma, PEFR is lower in the early morning hours. However, those with poor asthma control will exhibit a decline in PEFR throughout the day. There may be an exaggerated morning decrease of PEFR, and this is a very sensitive indicator of worsening airway inflammation and poor asthma control.

Simply monitoring the peak flow rate is unlikely to be of any value unless you have a clear understanding of what to do when this number suggests worsening airflow obstruction. For this purpose, some doctors recommend three color-coded PEFR zones to guide management. Others ask that patients call for help if peak flow decreases by 20 percent or more.

Other Tests for Respiratory Disorders

Blood Test Your doctor may get a sample of blood for a complete blood count and chemical profile. These results will help assess your general health and eliminate any

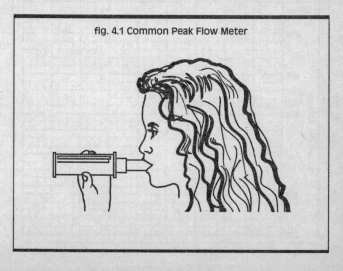

fig. 4.1 Common Peak Flow Meter

other disease as a possible cause of the respiratory problem. This test measures the amounts of red and white blood cells and shows how vital organs such as your kidney and liver are functioning. From the complete blood count, your doctor can tell whether you are anemic or have an infection. If you have serious lung disease with low oxygen levels in the blood, the red blood cell count may be high. An elevated red blood cell count may lead the doctor to do further investigations of oxygen levels and lung function to decide how to improve your condition.

Chest X Ray Although a chest X ray is not routinely required, if there are symptoms not explained by asthma, such as a cough productive of bloody sputum, your doc-

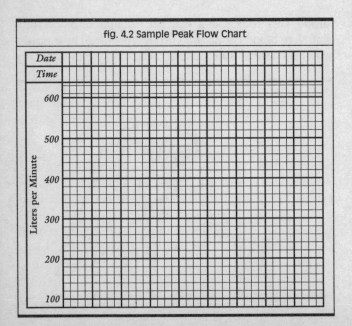

fig. 4.2 Sample Peak Flow Chart

tor may want this evaluation. Or, if you are not responding to the treatment regime, this test may help to clarify the problem.

Chest X rays usually show clear lungs for someone with asthma but may show various abnormalities if there is bronchiectasis, pneumonia, or other problems.

Computed Tomographic (CT) Scan A computed tomographic (CT or CAT) scan is a relatively expensive, special X-ray examination that is valuable for showing detailed images of the chest or sinuses when necessary to help explain the cause of various symptoms. It can show tumors, abnormal blood vessels, and infections in the lungs and can detect inflammation and obstruction in the sinuses. The CT scan involves a modest amount of radiation.

Electrocardiogram If you experience palpitations or chest pain with the breathing disorder, the doctor may order this test. Especially for those who are planning to begin an exercise program, this test will provide important information for the doctor. To make sure that your heart is not at risk during exertion, a cardiac stress test, including electrocardiography, may be suggested.

Methacholine Challenge Test After taking the spirometry test, your doctor may say that you have a normal expiratory flow of air. This does not *exclude* the possibility of asthma. Many of those with asthma have normal spirometry between attacks. The diagnosis of asthma in these individuals requires some form of bronchial irritation to induce airway obstruction.

If your doctor wants to do the methacholine test, this will usually be done in a pulmonary function laboratory. You will be asked to inhale a drug called methacholine in gradually increasing amounts. At each level of methacholine, spirometry will measure your breathing (page 69).

In a normal person, inhaling methacholine has almost no effect. However, if you have hyperreactivity of the bronchial tubes, methacholine will cause bronchoconstriction and result in a decrease in expiratory flows. While the test is generally safe and easy to do, you may experience minor wheezing and chest tightness after inhaling this drug, which may require the use of a bronchodilator for relief.

If the volume of air you can forcefully blow out in one second drops by 20 percent or more, and you also have episodes of shortness of breath, wheezing, or cough, this is certainly an indicator of asthma.

Oximetry or Arterial Blood Gases Oximetry is a noninvasive, painless method for measuring how much oxygen is in the arterial blood. A plastic probe containing a special light source and light meter is placed on your finger or earlobe. This will record the color of light reflected from the blood in that part of the body. The oximeter takes advantage of the fact that the color of the blood varies with the oxygen content. The higher the oxygen content, the redder the blood. The oximeter can correlate accurately the shade of the blood with its oxygen content.

In some people measuring carbon dioxide and oxygen levels in the blood is necessary. This requires obtaining a sample of arterial blood. Your doctor will use a small needle to puncture an artery to draw blood into a syringe. The blood will be analyzed in a special machine. Assessment of oxygenation and other blood gases such as carbon dioxide is sometimes important for diagnosis, as well as monitoring your response to treatment.

Paper Radioimmunosorbent Test (PRIST) The paper radioimmunosorbent test gives an accurate picture of the overall IgE level. IgE is an antibody that is bound to mast cells in the skin. A high level of this antibody can show if an allergy or infection is present. Following the levels of the IgE antibody is useful in assessing the response to treatment in certain cases of allergic disease. It must be emphasized that a normal level does not exclude the diagnosis of an allergic disease.

Purified Protein Derivative (PPD) Test This is a very helpful test for the diagnosis of tuberculosis and involves using the purified protein derivative from the bacteria that cause tuberculosis. A small amount of this preparation is injected into the skin on your forearm. A response showing that you were infected with TB includes a hardening of the skin where special cells that respond to the particular proteins congregate.

It is important to know that reactivity to PPD decreases with age. If an older person does not react to a first test, a repeat PPD skin test done one or two weeks later may be positive and considered significant of past infection.

Quantitative Immunoglobulin Determination Test The quantitative immunoglobulin determination test measures different immunoglobulin or antibody proteins in the blood. This test will give your doctor clues about your immune system. If certain levels are low, it is easier to become infected.

A sample of blood is obtained for the measurement of levels of immunoglobulin. If the IgE levels are high, your doctor might consider an allergic cause for symptoms such as rhinitis or asthma. If other specific immunoglobulins are increased in amount, then a certain infection may be suspected, such as pneumonia or a fungus. Decreased amounts of certain immunoglobulins may signal problems with the body's immune system defenses against certain infections caused by bacteria or viruses.

Radioallergosorbent Test (RAST) The radioallergosorbent test is a blood test used in detecting IgE reactions to specific triggers. It is done in a test tube. Although this test is no more accurate than skin tests, it may be considered for ultrasensitive persons for whom a skin test may pose a threat of a very severe allergic reaction. The RAST is more expensive than skin tests; however, it is not affected by medications you may be taking.

Skin Test Skin testing is suggested if there is a reasonable suspicion that a specific allergen or group of allergens is causing your symptoms. Skin tests involve injecting specific allergens under the skin to detect IgE mediated responses. If an allergen reacts with the IgE antibody, then histamine may be released. Your skin will respond with redness and swelling.

There are several types of skin tests your physician may use, including prick, intradermal, or patch. The most common is the prick method. Tiny drops of allergens are dropped on your skin, usually on the back. A needle is then pricked through the skin into each extract. Within a period of less than fifteen minutes, a hive will appear at the specific site if you have IgE antibodies to the particular allergen.

Sputum Examination Special tests of mucus from secretions in the nose and lungs can be helpful in making a diagnosis and determining the best manner of treatment. Your doctor will look for certain cells in the mucus that indicate allergic rhinitis or asthma may be the problem. Analyzing sputum coughed out of the lungs may also be helpful in diagnosing infections such as bacterial pneumonia or tuberculosis.

Developing a Personal Action Plan

Another step in getting back in control of your breathing problem and your life is to develop a *personal action plan*. This should be a collaborative effort between your primary physician, a specialist (allergist; ear, nose, and throat doctor; or pulmonologist) if you choose to use one, and your family members. In fact, family members should be encouraged to be involved in your treatment. Your physician may recommend special educational sessions for family members. Joint counseling for you and your family should also be available if needed.

Your pharmacist also plays a key role in providing education and information to help improve your quality of life. This health care professional can make sure you know both the brand names and the generic names of the medications being used, as well as the doses and common side effects of the various drugs. The pharmacist can report any problems to your prescribing physician.

Other key players in your personal action plan may include a registered/certified nutritionist to help with planning nutritional meals. A respiratory therapist can help with the various devices such as machines for delivering aerosol medications or oxygen and with the therapeutic processes needed for clearing secretion as in patients with bronchiectasis.

The plan you devise with your physician will be unique and fit your specific breathing and health needs. The main objective of this individualized plan is for you to stay active and healthy in spite of your chronic disease. As you learn more about your particular problem, begin to incorporate the following tips in your personal action plan to help manage the symptoms and prevent further damage.

Ten Tips to Help You Breathe Right Now

TIP 1: Avoid Cigarettes

Each year more than 390,000 people die of the effects of cigarette smoking. More than 3,000 of these deaths are from lung cancer directly attributable to tobacco smoke. While in the United States 1.5 million people quit smoking each year, as many as 50 million adults continue to smoke. Perhaps an even more disturbing statistic is that each day in the United States, more than 2,000 teenagers start to smoke for the first time. In fact, some revealing studies state that presently more than *one-third of all high school students* smoke cigarettes.

The problem arises as smoking greatly raises the risk of all types of health problems and is the major cause of emphysema, chronic bronchitis, and lung cancer. According to the American Lung Association, current male smokers over age thirty-five are ten times more likely to die of chronic obstructive pulmonary disease (COPD) and twenty-two times more likely to die of lung cancer than nonsmoking males. For women, lung cancer has now surpassed breast cancer as the leading cause of cancer deaths.

Tobacco smoke contains about 4,000 chemicals, including 200 known poisons. Not only does the smoker receive the health hazards of this destructive habit, but passive or secondhand smoke exposes innocent bystanders to poisons such as benzene, formaldehyde, and carbon monoxide. Sidestream smoke, the smoke you inhale from someone who is smoking, has even higher concentrations of some harmful poisons than mainstream smoke inhaled by the smoker. This passive smoking affects a nonsmoker's health and cause symptoms such as coughing, phlegm production, chest discomfort, and ultimately, reduced lung function.

The children of parents who smoke are greatly affected. More than 5,000 infants die annually from Sudden Infant Death Syndrome (SIDS), which is linked with maternal smoking. Secondhand cigarette smoke is also associated with an increased risk of lower respiratory tract infections, such as bronchitis and pneumonia. The U.S. Environmental Protection Agency estimates that 150,000 to 300,000 cases annually in infants and young children up to eighteen months of age are attributable to tobacco smoke. From 200,000 to 1 million children with asthma have their conditions worsened by exposure to cigarette smoke.

Though smoking increases the risk of respiratory problems and cancer, it is *one* important risk factor that you have control over. Although you cannot control the fact that you have two parents with asthma or that springtime blossoms cause allergy and sinusitis, *you can stop smoking.*

While it usually takes a serious disease to make one quit smoking, you can have a head start if you make a commitment today to stop. It must be recognized that cigarettes contain nicotine, a stimulant and addicting drug. After you stop smoking cigarettes, you may experience irritability, nervousness, and headaches for one to two weeks, especially if you have been a heavy smoker. The newer nonprescription nicotine patches that are worn on the skin, nicotine gum, or other medications can help you through the difficult period of withdrawal by making the physical problem less troublesome.

It is important to remember that even for those who have stopped smoking for years, the urge to smoke can always return. It is a matter of mental self-control to avoid cigarettes. Having the emotional support of a spouse, family, and understanding friends and coworkers is very important.

No matter how mild your respiratory problem, stopping smoking to reduce the risk of serious or even fatal breathing disorders is vital to your health. Soon after quitting, your ability to exercise will increase; even people who have smoked for years may notice an improvement in heart rate, blood pressure, and circulation to the hands, legs, and feet (see page 83). If you have trouble stopping, talk to your doctor or call your local chapter of the American Lung Association or the American Cancer Society.

TIP 2: Get It in Writing

Once you receive a proper diagnosis, it is important that your physician detail specific and personal instructions for treatment and prevention of further problems in writing. Your doctor may give you preprinted brochures or forms that outline the steps you are to take regarding medications, dosages, and timing. Information sheets that give a definition of your particular problem and how it can be managed should be available. Make sure your doctor or nurse shows you how to use any medication inhaler, and also a peak flow meter, and checks you on their use.

You may receive individualized forms to record the time and amount of medication you take along with any symptoms and medication response. This medication chart can help you keep track of the drug and doses. These forms can be brought to your next visit, and your doctor can see whether you are improving or whether you are using too much medication.

Have your doctor write down any emergency instructions. Ask for a detailed explanation of each medication needed for an emergency, such as an Epi-Pen (epinephrine) for anaphylactic reactions. Write down emergency numbers and also the numbers of family and close friends who might help you during an episode.

When Smokers Quit

Within twenty minutes of smoking that last cigarette, the body begins a series of changes that continues for years.

20 MINUTES
Blood pressure drops to normal.
Pulse rate drops to normal.
Body temperature of hands and feet increases to normal.

8 HOURS
Carbon monoxide level in blood drops to normal.
Oxygen level in blood increases to normal.

24 HOURS
Chance of heart attack decreases.

48 HOURS
Nerve endings start regrowing.
Ability to smell and taste is enhanced.

2 WEEKS TO 3 MONTHS
Circulation improves.
Walking becomes easier.
Lung function increases up to 30 percent.

1 TO 9 MONTHS
Coughing, sinus congestion, fatigue, and shortness of breath decrease.
Cilia regrow in lungs; this increases the ability to handle mucus, clean

1 TO 9 MONTHS (CONT.)
the lungs, and reduce infection.
Body's overall energy increases.

1 YEAR
Excess risk of coronary heart disease is half that of a smoker.

5 YEARS
Lung cancer death rate for average former smoker (one pack a day) decreases by almost half.
Stroke risk is reduced to that of a nonsmoker five to fifteen years after quitting.
Risk of cancer in the mouth, throat, and esophagus decreases to half that of a smoker.

10 YEARS
Lung cancer death rate is similar to that of nonsmokers.
Precancerous cells are replaced.
Risk of cancer to mouth, throat, esophagus, bladder, kidney, and pancreas decreases.

15 YEARS
Risk of coronary heart disease is that of a nonsmoker.

SOURCE: American Cancer Society and the National Centers for Disease Control and Prevention.

TIP 3: Identify the Triggers

As you gain insight into your particular illness, it is important to understand the triggers that set you up for such episodes as a sinus infection, wheezing or cough, shortness of breath, and runny nose. These triggers can be *allergens* (pollens, molds, pet dander, dust mites), *irritants* (smoke, chemical sprays, odors), and *physical changes* (cold air, weather fronts, exercise). Removing the trigger is vital to controlling respiratory problems. In fact, avoiding common household and environmental allergens is one of the best ways to lessen many problems.

When you come in contact with a trigger, do not think that symptoms will be alleviated on their own. It is important to have symptom-controlling medication, as described in Chapter 5, with you always and use any preventive and reliever measures your doctor has described. If possible, avoid known triggers or reduce their effects quickly.

Chapter 6 gives proactive avoidance and environmental control measures to help you begin a personal action program to allergy-proof your home and workplace.

TIP 4: Know Your Early Warning Signs

When your problem is worsening, you will probably experience such problems as wheezing, coughing, sneezing, shortness of breath, fatigue, achiness, headache, ear pain, sinus pain, runny or stuffy nose, chin or throat itchiness, dark circles under the eyes, or difficulty sleeping. Being aware of these signs and symptoms is important, along with noticing any changes on your peak flow meter, if asthma or COPD is your problem. Use the warning signs and symptoms listed in Chapters 2 and 3 to assess other respiratory problems. For example, such emergency warning signs as rapid or shallow breathing, inability to breathe deeply, or a bluish tinge to fingernails and lips could signal respiratory distress and mandate immediate medical attention.

TIP 5: Take Correct Medications and Proper Doses

Metered dose inhalers or oral medications are a vital part of your personal action plan. These medications have been prescribed specifically for your problem. Whether it is an inhaler, a saline spray, oral decongestants, antibiotics, or steroids, take the medication or breathing treatment as directed for the best management of your problem.

Avoid taking over-the-counter medications—without first consulting your physician. There are a myriad of over-the-counter medications—some helpful and some not so helpful. If you are taking an over-the-counter decongestant or antihistamine, be sure to ask your doctor whether it will help your symptoms, not worsen them. Some medications such as aspirin or nonsteroid anti-inflammatory medications like ibuprofen can worsen symptoms for many with asthma and allergy.

TIP 6: Keep a Symptom Diary

Keeping a daily diary along with a symptom account can help you in tracking your breathing problems and finding reasonable solutions. In this diary, you should keep track of any symptoms, along with your peak flow rate, twice daily. All medications, including over-the-counter medications, should be recorded, as should any side effects that are unusual.

Writing down known triggers that are causing your breathing problems is also important. For example, you may write in your diary that you have difficulty breathing and feel fatigued after stressful times at home or work. Or, you may note that you experienced new symptoms after walking by the perfume counter at the department store. Weeks later when you look back on these dates, you can see a pattern between the increase in your respiratory symptoms and possible triggers.

Perhaps you find that you have not slept well in days. Reading your diary will enable you to identify problems such as nocturnal asthma, a chest cold, or chronic sinus headaches you may have had that contributed to the sleep problems.

While you are taking medications, keep a record of symptoms and list the treatments you tried and how effective they were. If you are allergic to certain foods, keeping track of your daily diet and allergic symptoms can be lifesaving.

Sharing this diary with your physician at your next visit is important. It may help in prescribing more effective medications that will enable you to continue doing the things you enjoy.

TIP 7: Engage in Regular Exercise and Activity

Exercise and physical conditioning are important parts of a personal action plan to manage most chronic diseases. Regular activity will allow you to strengthen your respiratory muscles and improve your overall fitness; this can help boost your immune system—the body's defense against infection—and ward off other illness. Exercise also helps generate adrenaline, which helps constrict swollen blood vessels and relieve nasal stuffiness.

If you have symptoms that cause you to avoid or even fear exercise, talk with your doctor about medications that can be taken before and during exercise to allow you to function at a normal level. If your symptoms are still not controlled, ask for a referral to a respiratory therapist who can show you how to do pursed lip breathing and specific exercises to help strengthen respiratory muscles and clear out phlegm by effective coughing. Pulmonary rehabilitation which includes the input of a respiratory therapist can enable you to stay more active and enjoy life.

TIP 8: Eat Nutritious Foods

Meal planning that includes plenty of nutritious foods each day is important to maintain good health and immune function. Chapter 8 gives you insight into the healing power of phytochemicals and antioxidants which are important for boosting immune function for those with respiratory problems.

Congestion, shortness of breath, excess mucus production, scratchy or swollen throat, and overall fatigue can often diminish appetite. Talk with a registered nutritionist/dietitian for help in your particular case, and be sure your diet is full of healing nutrients. It is also important to get to your ideal body weight. Obesity increases the work of the respiratory muscles and the heart.

TIP 9: Reduce Stress

Some complementary stress reduction techniques suggested in Chapter 11 are important to help keep your life and disease in perspective and deal with any breathing problem in a more reasonable manner.

As you take proactive steps to reduce stress and increase recovery, don't ignore your need for rest and sleep. Rest is particularly important as it enables the body to heal. If you are having sleep difficulties, see Chapter 9 for some helpful and practical suggestions.

Worry and anxiety will only exacerbate your problem. Especially if you are having difficulty breathing, it is important to know ahead of time how to get medical help quickly, including how to call for emergency help if needed. Have someone available who can take you to the emergency room. If you have difficulty breathing that is not relieved with medication, take immediate action with a call to your physician or a trip to the emergency room. Emergency care is warranted if breathing becomes labored and you are struggling to catch your breath. If you are unsure, go anyway to be safe.

TIP 10: Maintain a Positive Attitude

Keeping a positive attitude with a chronic breathing disorder may be hard. The inability to catch your breath at times can make you feel sorry for yourself and cause other emotional problems. Nevertheless, one of the most powerful weapons you have is a strong, positive attitude. Your outlook on life and on your well-being is free and has no side effects. Many physicians will attest to the fact that the patients with chronic illnesses who have the best chance for recovery are those with an upbeat and positive attitude.

Although the goal in most cases of breathing disorders is not for a cure, it is reasonable to expect to be able to control the symptoms and enjoy better breathing. This means that you should start feeling better, experience fewer symptoms, and decrease episodes of congestion or shortness of breath. You should expect to get around and do the things you would like to do in reasonable comfort. The good news is that most people can improve. It is very unusual to see persons who cannot be helped at all, even with years of inflamed airways and infections.

Tips for Your Personal Action Plan

1. Avoid cigarettes.
2. Get it in writing.
3. Identify the triggers.
4. Know your early warning signs.
5. Take correct medications and proper doses.
6. Keep a symptom diary.
7. Engage in regular exercise and activity.
8. Eat nutritious foods.
9. Reduce stress.
10. Maintain a positive attitude.

Regain Your Life

Following the ten tips for your personal action plan will enable you to approach breathing problems in a positive way. Because of new technology and understanding of respiratory problems, your confusing combination of symptoms along with loss of activity can now be accurately diagnosed. As you methodically make specific lifestyle changes for better breathing, you will find yourself back in control of your life and health.

Read on and continue to learn how to manage your breathing problem in an orderly manner. However, keep in mind that while this resource guide gives you the latest information you need, each person is different. Talk with your doctor for specific advice about your own situation, and then follow the many suggestions outlined in this book. Join those persons who have learned to manage their breathing problems and are enjoying life again.

chapter 5

Selecting Medical Treatment

A myriad of medical options are now available to prevent and treat breathing disorders. Although these usually provide no cures for the problems, they can give much-needed relief of the various symptoms without causing harmful side effects. Usually, the treatment measures can halt the disease, and so prevent further damage and deterioration.

Compared with treatment methods used a century ago, today's medical options might be considered miraculous. In *Mornings on Horseback*, the dramatic story of Theodore Roosevelt's childhood years and his personal suffering with asthma, author David McCullough presents a graphic picture of the treatment of asthma in the 1870s.

The common methods then used to confront an attack varied greatly and to the present-day reader seem excessively harsh. Emetics and purges were standard. The common way to avert an attack was to make the patient violently ill, to dose him with ipecac or with incredibly nauseating potions made of garlic and mustard seed and "vinegar of squills," a dried plant also used for rat poison. Children were given enemas, plunged into cold baths. Whiskey and gin were used, laudanum (opium mixed with wine) and Indian hemp (marijuana). The patient was made to inhale chloroform or the fumes of burning nitrate paper or the smoke from dried jimson weed (Datura stramonium), another poisonous plant, coarse and vile smelling, that had been used in treating asthma in India for centuries. Many children were made to smoke a ghastly medicinal cigarette concocted of jimson weed and chopped camphor.

Black coffee may have been the Roosevelts' "trump card," . . . but Teedie (Theodore Roosevelt) was also made to swallow ipecac and smoke cigars. The purpose of the cigar was to subject the child to what, in essence, was a dose of nicotine poisoning. "In those who have not established a tolerance to tobacco," explained Henry Hyde Salter (an English physician at that time and author of the book *On Asthma*), "its use is soon followed by a well-known condition of collapse, much resembling sea-sickness—vertigo, loss of power in the limbs, a sense of deadly faintness, cold sweat, inability to speak or think, nausea, vomiting."

Imagine your child or anyone for that matter having to smoke a cigar until he or she vomited to find relief for respiratory congestion! There is no question that researchers have come a long way in providing control and relief for most breathing problems.

Liz, a sixteen-year-old high school junior, has had allergies and asthma since she was in second grade. Although she suffered with ear infections and food allergies as a preschooler, it was not until she had the flu at age seven when she was diagnosed with asthma.

Since that time almost ten years ago, Liz and her mother have spent hundreds of hours and thousands of dollars with many different allergy, asthma, and pulmonary specialists. They have searched for safe, effective treatments to open Liz's inflamed airways and to allow her to have a normal childhood and adolescence. Liz's bathroom cabinet is filled with the results of this search—a colorful collection of various inhaled bronchodilator cases, anti-inflammatory inhalers, decongestant syrups, antihistamine pills, bronchodilator tablets, and her trusty peak flow meter.

About two years ago, a physician friend told Liz's mother about a new inhaled medicine, salmeterol (Serevent), that had shown great promise for many people with asthma. Salmeterol is especially useful for people like Liz who continue to depend on short-acting inhaled beta2-agonists four to six times a day, as well as anti-inflammatory therapy using oral or inhaled steroids. It can also help those whose sleep is disturbed by nighttime symptoms. Furthermore, a single dose (two puffs) of salmeterol prevents exercise-induced bronchospasm for *up to twelve hours*.

Realizing that salmeterol was not to be used for an acute attack, Liz started on this long-acting medication, and it virtually changed her life. Instead of planning her life around her asthma and medications, Liz was able to focus on her many activities and friends. Rather than her asthma controlling her, she now controls the disease, using the new long-acting inhaler twice a day, before school and at bedtime, along with an inhaled steroid.

We share true stories like this one not to give false hope or to replace recommendations by your doctor. They are told to inform you of the latest treatments and how these can work for many as part of a successful management program.

Do the measures work for everyone? While we cannot guarantee that the treatment and prevention measures will solve your specific problem, we do know that these medicines allow millions of people to get back in control of their breathing problem. Use this information to talk with your doctor as you seek professional advice that meets your particular respiratory needs.

A Stepwise Approach

Your doctor is crucial to good control of your breathing disorder. However, continue to keep in mind that *you* are also a vital, active participant. The ultimate goal is to control or manage the problem, and only you can accurately follow your physician's recommendations.

A stepwise approach to therapy recommends that the number and frequency of medications are increased with the escalating severity of your disease. This selection is also made on the basis of your age and other health concerns, current treatment, pharmacologic properties, availability of treatment, and economic considerations.

Remember that the choice of medication depends on the judgment of a skilled, experienced physician. Follow-up is essential to gauge the response to the treatment and to make changes as needed. Use the following information to see what successful options you can use to breathe better.

Allergy and Nasal Problems

A red, swollen, and constantly dripping nose can make anyone irritable. As you may have experienced, finding the right type relief for allergy and nasal congestion is important. Sometimes it is difficult to find that perfect medication that works effectively but has no side effects, such as fatigue or nervousness.

Many medicines that have a positive *effect* on your ailment, can also affect your body in a less than positive manner. For example, decongestants can give optimal relief for a swollen, congested nose. Yet the side effects of insomnia or nervousness are often a difficult trade-off. That is why understanding the purpose, ingredients, and specific warnings for each type of medication is important to your overall health as well as your swollen nasal passages. When you can find that right medicine that clears up symptoms yet allows you to live a healthy, normal life, then you will feel in control of your problem.

While there is no quick fix for your runny or congested nose, antihistamines and decongestants continue to be the two most widely used forms of treatment for allergic rhinitis, colds, sinusitis, and a host of other respiratory problems. If an infection is involved, antibiotics are still the standard mode of treatment, and these differ greatly. If you are allergic to penicillin, your doctor should be aware of this as other highly effective antibiotics are available. There are also generic brands or name brands, some that are equally effective and some that are not.

You may find excellent relief with short-term decongestant, saline, or steroid nasal sprays that can significantly reduce the swelling in your nasal passage and sinuses and help to ease the problem. *Expectorants* are useful if your mucus is thick and hard to expel. This medicine liquefies mucus so it drains easily; this can help reduce swelling and pain.

The most important key is to understand the treatment, including the effect and side effects, and then trust your doctor to make the best decision with your overall health in mind.

Antihistamines

Antihistamines have been taken safely by millions of allergic people for more than fifty years. Although these medications do *not* cure your allergy or congestion, they do block the effect of histamine and help relieve such annoying symptoms as sneezing, itching, congestion, and discharge, and also other skin and eye conditions.

Your doctor may prescribe short-acting antihistamines, taken every four to six hours, or timed-release antihistamines, taken every twelve hours. On the basis of scientific evidence, we know that these drugs work best if taken *before* symptoms begin. In this regard, the medications can build up in the blood if taken regularly for three to four days to give a protective effect.

The most common side effects of antihistamines are sedation, drowsiness, and dry mouth. You may want to take any sedating antihistamine at night before bedtime to avoid feeling sluggish during the day. Some prescription antihistamines, such as terfenadine (Seldane), can be taken during the day without drowsiness. There are new reports that when Seldane is combined with an antibiotic, such as erythromycin or ketocanazole, it can cause very dangerous abnormal rhythms of the heart. Consequently, it is being reevaluated for its safety. Newer antihistamines such as loratadine (Claritin), fexofenadine (Allegra), and certirizine (Zyrtec) are also highly effective and unlikely to cause drowsiness or deleterious side effects.

Antihistamines have *no* role in the treatment of sinusitis as they can cause drying of mucous membranes and interfere with the clearing of secretions. However, they are useful for your allergy symptoms as previously suggested.

Brand Names of Common Antihistamines	
OVER THE COUNTER	PRESCRIPTION
Benadryl	Allegra
Chlor-Trimeton	Claritin
Dimetane	Hismanal
Tavist	Seldane
	Zyrtec

Decongestants

If you live with constantly swollen nasal passages from allergic rhinitis, a cold, or sinusitis, decongestants are the medication of choice. Nasal decongestants that are taken orally come in many forms, such as pills, tablets, capsules, or syrups. They are used to open the mucous membranes in the nose and help them drain.

Commonly used decongestants include phenyl-propanolamine, pseudoephedrine, and phenylephrine. All these work the same way to reduce swelling and congestion. These agents may be found alone or more frequently in combination with other medications under many brand names (see the box "Brand Names of Common Decongestants").

With a decongestant, you may experience insomnia or nervousness. To decrease these effects, try taking only the morning dose. Avoid these medications if you have severe hypertension, coronary artery disease, or take certain psychiatric medications such as Parnate, a monamine oxidase inhibitor (MAO) used to treat severe depression. If you have hyperthyroidism, diabetes mellitus, or prostate disease, only use these medications with your doctor's consent.

Nasal Sprays

If you need *immediate relief* for a swollen, congested nasal passage, decongestant nasal sprays such as oxymetazoline (Afrin) and phenylephrine (Neo-Synephrine) can be helpful. Unlike oral decongestants, it is important to stop using decongestant nasal sprays after three to five days to avoid the development of rebound congestion or recurrent congestion (see the box "Common Nasal Steroid Sprays"). Most of the sprays carry a warning, which should be read before usage.

Brand Names of Common Nasal Decongestants	
Afrin	Ornex
Allerest	Sinarest
Comtrex	Sine-Off
Dristan	Sinutab
Neosynephrine	Sudafed

Antibiotics

The standard treatment for upper and lower respiratory infections is an antibiotic. The antibiotic will get to the root of the problem, which is usually infection caused by bacteria. An antibiotic is used if you have an increased amount of thick mucus or mucus that is colored (yellow, green, or brown).

In adults, it can take several days for antibiotics to work on sinus infections because of the rather poor blood supply in the sinuses. However, if you do not find relief within a few days for any respiratory tract infection, check back with your doctor to see whether the antibiotic is working for your particular infection. Certain bacteria have become resistant to some antibiotics in some locales, and stronger medications may be needed.

Generally, the duration of antibiotic therapy treatment is ten to fourteen days, but may be longer in cases of chronic sinusitis. Some newer antibiotics require a shorter duration of therapy. If treatment with medicine does not produce a relief of symptoms or adequate drainage, it may be necessary to check with your physician for more treatment measures.

The selection of an antibiotic depends on careful assessment by your doctor, who will decide which antibiotic is the most helpful, depending on your diagnosis and then prescribe the safest, most effective, and least costly drug or combination of drugs. It is important to notify your doctor of any side effects experienced such as a skin rash, increased breathing problems, or other symptoms.

Nasal Steroids

Because inflammation is a key sign of allergy and nasal problems, inhaled nasal steroids can give good relief. These prescription medications help prevent or reduce inflammation in the nasal passages and sinuses when exposed to a specific allergen (pollen, animal dander, or dust mites). The spray is placed inside the nose and used one or more times a day. Some sprays are liquid; others are aerosol puffs.

Antibiotics Frequently Used for Respiratory Infections	
BRAND NAME	GENERIC NAME
Amoxil	Amoxicillin
Augmentin	Amoxicillin-potassium clavulanate
Biaxin	Clarithromycin
Bactrim, Septra	Trimethoprim-sulfamethoxazole
Ceclor	Cefaclor
Cipro	Ciprofloxacin
Floxin	Ofloxacin
Omnipen	Ampicillin
Pen-Vee K	Penicillin and potassium
Sumycin	Tetracycline
Vibramycin	Doxycycline
Zithromax	Azithromycin

It is important to note that you will *not* find immediate relief with the steroid sprays. In time, they will help decrease mucus production. Your doctor may want you to continue other medications to reduce inflammation until the maximum effect is felt with the steroid spray, usually after one to two weeks. In some cases of seasonal allergic rhinitis, the other medication(s) may need to be used for longer periods of time.

For rhinitis associated with a drippy, nasal discharge,

ipratropium bromide (Atrovent nasal) may be very effective. This medication helps to reduce nasal discharge.

Nasal Wash

Nasal saline solutions are used to restore moisture to your sinuses and may help lessen inflamed nasal membranes. If used regularly, they can help decrease postnasal drip and cleanse your passages of bacteria. These agents are mild and safe to use. Over-the-counter nasal saline sprays include Ocean and NaSal sprays.

Common Nasal Steroid Sprays	
BRAND NAME	GENERIC NAME
Beconase, Beconase AQ	Beclomethasone
Flonase	Fluticasone
Nasacort	Triamcinolone
Nasalide	Flunisolide
Rhinocort	Budesonide
Vancenase, Vancenase AQ	Beclomethasone

A word of caution: Too frequent and overly prolonged usage of any nasal spray or wash may cause counterproductive irritation and actually worsen or cause problems of congestion or drip.

Drugs Affecting Mucus

A *mucokinetic agent* is a drug that helps thin mucus to make it easier to flow. Many experts feel that water is the most beneficial medium to help liquefy mucus; you can also use such medications as guaifenesin (Robitussin Expectorant or HumiBid). Make sure the expectorant does not contain an antihistamine or cough suppressants unless prescribed by your doctor. The most frequent adverse effect of expectorants is nausea and vomiting.

Asthma and Other Lung Diseases

Most of the medical treatments you will use for asthma and other obstructive lung diseases are the same. Although there are suggested drugs for the various diseases, your treatment will be individualized, according to your specific disease, symptoms, and health status. Many medications for asthma and lung diseases fall into two categories:

Anti-inflammatory medications
Bronchodilators

Controller or Reliever

Medications for asthma and other lung diseases are classified as *controller* and *reliever* medications. The anti-inflammatory medications are the controllers and keep symptoms at bay. The beta2-agonist medications are the relievers for most cases of acute bronchospasm. The primary action of the beta2-agonists is to relax bronchial smooth muscles. Because beta2-agonists do not have any anti-inflammatory action, these drugs have no role in *prevention* of acute exacerbation. Doesn't it make sense to try to prevent attacks from occurring at all?

Inhaled, Oral, or Intravenous

You can take medications for asthma and other lung diseases in different ways, including by inhaling, orally, and intravenously. Inhaling medicine is typically the best way as the drug goes straight into the airways and side effects are decreased. Also, inhaled bronchodilators will help relieve your symptoms much faster than oral medication.

Inhaled medicines can be delivered into your system in a variety of ways, including:

Metered dose inhalers (MDIs)

Dry powder inhalers
Nebulized aerosols

A metered dose inhaler (MDI) delivers medication through a small, handheld aerosol canister. You do not breathe into the canister; rather, the MDI puffs the medicine into your lungs when you press down on the inhaler.

The dry powder inhaler requires you to breathe in deeply as the medication enters your lungs. This may be difficult for some as a minimal inspiratory flow rate is necessary to inhale the medication. It may also be difficult to use this type inhaler during an asthma attack when you cannot fully catch a deep breath.

Nebulized aerosols, which forcefully deliver inhaled medication deep into the lungs are useful for children under age five or if you are unable to inhale from an MDI. The nebulizer uses a small spraylike instrument to change the liquid medication or saline solution into a fine mist. When you hold the face mask or mouthpiece up to your lips and turn on the compression machine, the nebulizer helps the delivery into your lungs. This type inhaled medication can be a lifesaver during an acute episode.

No matter which type inhaler you choose, ask your doctor for specific instructions and make sure your technique is checked regularly.

Spacers

If you have trouble finding relief with a metered dose inhaler, a *spacer*, or *holding chamber*, will help improve the delivery of the medicine. A spacer is especially helpful if you have difficulty coordinating your breathing and spraying. Two commonly used spacers are Inspirease and AeroChamber.

To use a spacer, first blow into it to make sure it is free of debris. Your inhaler is then pushed into one end of the spacer; the other end is placed between your teeth. When you puff your inhaler, the medication goes inside the tube where it is held in a reservoir. Then it can be inhaled leisurely into your lungs. This method helps to space out large drops of medicine that frequently do not even reach your airways.

The benefits of using a spacer to deliver inhaled medicines are tremendous. Some studies have found that *without* a spacer, as much as *90 percent* of inhaled medication does not even enter the lungs! The spacer can also help to reduce sore mouth, cough, hoarseness, and thrush. Thrush is a fungal infection that can occur with the use of corticosteroids. It looks like creamy-white, curdlike patches in the mouth and is treated with an antifungal drug.

How to Use a Metered Dose Inhaler*

1. Hold the inhaler upright and shake.
2. Remove the cap.
3. With your head tilted back, exhale normally.
4. Place the inhaler about 1 to 2 inches from your mouth.
5. Press down on the inhaler's canister while inhaling. Be sure to keep your mouth open and breathe in for five seconds.
6. Hold your breath for ten seconds longer.
7. Repeat the steps depending on how many puffs you are prescribed.

*The preferred way to use an inhaler is with a spacer.

Corticosteroids (Steroids)

Steroids are very valuable in the treatment of asthma, as well as other lung diseases. Steroids are anti-inflammatory medications that reduce mucus production in the airways and prevent swelling of the mucousal membranes. If you ever had a serious asthma attack or problems with COPD, you may have had high doses of steroids administered intravenously in the hospital. Using this principle, short-term use of steroids for reducing inflammation is very effective in improving breathing in most respiratory diseases. When used in a severe attack, no doubt the benefits of steroids far outweigh the risks.

Oral

A brief course of oral steroids, usually for two weeks, may be used when your symptoms worsen but you do not require hospitalization. Your doctor might prescribe prednisone (Deltasone) or methylprednisolone (Medrol). While a two-week course, or "short burst," of steroids is relatively safe, try to avoid steroids on a long-term basis as there are serious side effects (see page 104). Taking supplemental calcium at this time may help you to prevent osteoporosis or thinning of the bones, which is one serious side effect of long-term steroid use. If you need steroids frequently for "rescue" therapy, this can suggest poor control of airway inflammation or continued exposure to some unsuspected allergen. In this case, talk to your doctor about newer inhaled medications.

Inhaled

In asthma and some cases of COPD, inhaled steroids can be used effectively in place of low-dose oral steroids. Commonly used inhaled steroids include triamcinolone (Azmacort), flunisolide (Aerobid), beclomethasone (Vanceril or Beclovent), and fluticasone (Flovent). These have proven to become the first line treatment for asthma and may play a role in other lung diseases. In fact, recent studies support the use of inhaled steroids early in the course of disease. After introduction of inhaled steroids, the need for oral steroids may decrease.

Unlike the serious side effects of oral steroids, the most

common side effects of inhaled steroids are hoarseness and thrush, especially in elderly adults. You should rinse the mouth carefully and gargle with water after inhalation to help reduce the risk of oral thrush. The lowest dose required to control and prevent symptoms should be used.

Mast Cell Stabilizer

Prevention of symptoms is crucial with any disease. A type of medication called a mast cell stabilizer may *prevent* allergic reactions.

Common Side Effects Associated with Oral Steroid Therapy
Suppression of adrenal glands Osteoporosis or thinning of the bones Diabetes Retention of fluid and salt Hypertension Weight gain Myopathy, or deterioration of the muscles Psychiatric disturbances Skin fragility Cataracts Frequent infections

In the nasal passage, a spray called cromolyn sodium (Nasalcrom) is effective in blocking the allergy response and is used even when you are symptom-free. Nasalcrom used to be available by prescription only but now is available over the counter. Ask your doctor whether it would work in your situation.

Cromolyn Sodium

Inhaled cromolyn sodium is also effective if you have allergic asthma or exercise-induced asthma (EIA). However, compared with inhaled steroids, this mast cell stabilizer is less potent.

Although the exact mechanisms of how it works are still unknown, the main advantage of cromolyn sodium is its excellent track record of safety and lack of side effects. Consequently, many pediatricians prefer to employ cromolyn sodium over inhaled steroids as first-line controller medications in children. However, for adults, there is no reason you should choose cromolyn sodium over inhaled steroids to control airway inflammation.

Nedocromil Sodium

Although nedocromil sodium (Tilade) is chemically unrelated to cromolyn sodium, this newer inhaled medication has very similar actions, especially with asthma and EIA. Some preliminary studies even suggest that nedocromil sodium may have some steroid-like, anti-inflammatory benefit. If you fail to achieve adequate asthma control despite a combined use of inhaled steroids and theophylline, a trial of inhaled nedocromil sodium may be helpful.

Inhaled Beta2-agonists

Short-acting beta2-agonists such as albuterol (Proventil, Ventolin) that are inhaled are the therapies of choice for the *relief of acute bronchospasm* with most diseases of the lung. Using this medicine before exercise or anticipated exposure to a known trigger may block the development of acute symptoms. However, if you use this drug round the clock for an extended period of time, it may lead to the development of tolerance. This causes a reduction in the medicine's effect and shortens its duration of action. You are encouraged to use this inhaler only on an as-needed basis. For rescue or rapid relief, Proventil HFA containing alhaterol without the chlorofluorocarbon propellant is now available with a newly designed delivery system that is more dependable than the older version.

A *longer acting* inhaled beta2-agonist called salmeterol (Serevent) is now helping many people with asthma and even some with other diseases such as COPD. This inhaler is used only twice a day (two puffs each time). Unlike the short-acting inhaled beta2-agonist, which is a *reliever medication* for acute attacks, salmeterol is a *controller medication*. Its effect on the airways is not immediate and should never be used in an acute attack.

Common Side Effects of Beta2-agonists
Dizziness
Fast or pounding heartbeat
Increased systolic blood pressure
Nervousness
Tremors

Ipratropium Bromide

If you are a middle-aged or older adult with asthma, emphysema, or chronic bronchitis, regular use of an inhaled medication called ipratropium (Atrovent) may be helpful. Although any-aged person can use this, it seems to work best in adults over forty.

How does it work? In your body, the *vagus nerve* affects airway muscle tone and mucus secretion. When the vagus nerve is stimulated, acetylcholine is produced (see page 223). This chemical contracts the airway muscle and causes mucus stimulation. Ipratropium blocks the action of acetylcholine.

Ipratropium has a slower onset and longer action than beta2-agonists like albuterol. Many sufferers find good control using it along with a beta2-agonist (up to four times a day). Side effects can include dryness of mouth, cough, nervousness, headache, palpitations, and blurring of vision if sprayed near the eyes. Combivent (a combination of albuterol and ipratropium) is now available.

Theophylline

Theophylline, a relatively weak bronchodilator, is a chemical similar to caffeine. It may stimulate the heart, the central nervous system, and the skeletal muscles, while also relaxing the smooth muscles, including the airway muscles.

Theophylline had been the first choice for asthma and lung disease therapy for nearly five decades. However, with the newer inhaled steroids and increased reports about theophylline toxicity, there is a decrease in its use. Nonetheless, if inhaled steroids do not work for your situation, your doctor may prescribe it with good results. It is often used with toddlers and preschool children who cannot use inhaled steroids. When taken at bedtime, it may control nighttime symptoms.

If you have COPD, theophylline may play an even greater role in treatment, especially if you cannot use inhaled medicines. Also, if you are not responding satisfactorily to the combination of ipratropium (Atrovent) and albuterol (Ventolin), your doctor may add theophylline to your medications. Used in this manner, theophylline can improve respiratory muscle function, stimulate the respiratory center, and enhance the activities of daily living.

An extra bonus of using theophylline as a bronchodilator is that it helps to expel mucus, an important effect for those with COPD, and to strengthen the diaphragm, the main inspiratory muscle.

Some of the popular brand names of oral theophylline include Respbid, Slo-bid, Theo-dur, Theo-24, and Uniphyl. Many illnesses and commonly prescribed drugs reduce the clearance of theophylline from the body. This increases the risk of serious toxicity. If you use this drug, make sure your doctor monitors you closely and have your theophylline level checked periodically by means of a blood test.

Common Side Effects of Theophylline	
Abnormal heart rhythms	Nausea
Diarrhea	Seizures*
Fast, pounding heart beat	Stomachache
Headache	Vomiting
Insomnia	
Irritability	*This may occur during over-
Muscle twitching	dose when blood levels are
	excessively high.

Common Illnesses and Drugs That Increase the Theophylline Level and the Risk of Toxicity
ILLNESSES
Heart disease
Hypothyroidism
Liver disease
Pneumonia
Sustained high fever
Viral upper respiratory infections
DRUGS
Alcohol (in drinks and some medications)
Allopurinol
Cimetidine (in Tagamet for digestive problems)
Antibiotics (ciprofloxacin and erythromycin)
Estrogen hormones (used in oral contraceptives)
Propranolol (beta blocker used for hypertension)
Verapamil (calcium channel blocker used for hypertension)
Methotrexate (an immunosuppressant drug)
SPECIAL CONDITIONS
Obesity
Stopping cigarette smoking

Immunosuppressive Therapy

Some people find that even with long-term oral steroid use, their symptoms stay unmanaged and out of control. If you have experienced this, you may be in the minority of people who are *steroid resistant*. Your doctor may then try an immunosuppressive drug such as methotrexate. Immunosuppressive drugs have serious toxicity, so be sure this therapy has the close medical supervision of an expert experienced in the use of these medications.

Newer Drugs: Leukotriene Inhibitors and Antagonists

Be sure to ask your doctor about some breakthrough drugs on the market used for asthma and other lung diseases. One such drug is zafirlukast (Accolate), which is now on the pharmacists' shelves. This drug works at the level of the cell receptors which ordinarily respond to leukotrienes. *Leukotrienes* are substances released from the membranes of mast cells during IgE-mediated reactions and cause the uncomfortable bronchoconstriction and excessive secretion of mucus. Zafirlukast (Accolate) keeps bronchial tubes from constricting. Some researchers have found that this new type medication may be almost as effective as steroids without the side effects.

Oxygen Therapy

Oxygen therapy is being used more frequently for many lung diseases. This is likely due to a combination of an aging population, an increased prevalence of patients with COPD, and the knowledge that oxygen is necessary to have a good quality of life.

If you are short of breath, this does not necessarily mean that oxygen will be prescribed as you may not benefit. Rather, your doctor may prescribe oxygen when your level of oxygen in the blood has been measured and is abnormally low. It is only at this time that oxygen will offer a benefit. Two landmark studies, including the Nocturnal Oxygen Therapeutic Trial in 1980 in North America and the Medical Research Council study in 1981 in England, reported that people with abnormally low oxygen levels increased their survival by using supplementary oxygen. Even those who used oxygen for part of the day (twelve to fifteen hours a day) improved survival. However, as these studies showed, using continuous oxygen around the clock gives even better survival statistics than the noncontinuous use of oxygen.

Controller and Reliever Medications

CONTROLLERS, *MEDICATIONS TAKEN DAILY TO KEEP PERSISTENT SYMPTOMS UNDER CONTROL*

Inhaled corticosteroids
Systemic corticosteroids
Cromolyn sodium
Nedocromil sodium
Sustained release theophylline
Long-acting inhaled beta2-agonists
Immunosuppressive drugs
Leukotriene inhibitors or antagonists

RELIEVERS, *MEDICATIONS USED TO RELIEVE BRONCHOCONSTRICTION AND ACUTE SYMPTOMS*

Short-acting inhaled beta2-agonists
Systemic corticosteroids (especially intravenous)
Short-acting theophylline

When speaking about low oxygen levels, it is important to discuss air travel. This is sometimes a challenge for those with respiratory problems, particularly COPD, as newer aircraft cruise at very high altitudes. The cabin pressure inside the plane is only able to partially correct the change in atmospheric pressure. If you have COPD, you may find yourself on a plane and experience what it is like to inhale air at 9,000-foot (2,743-meter) altitude. One study showed that two-thirds of those with severe COPD had arterial oxygen levels that were significantly reduced below safe ranges after forty-five minutes at 2,438 meters!

Although the prevalence of in-flight low oxygen levels and related medical problems and deaths is not accurately known, common sense tells you to take precautions ahead of time. Formulas have been developed using the oxygen level in the blood at sea level along with the forced expiratory volume in one second to predict fairly accurately the level of oxygen in the blood at altitude. If the level of oxygen in your blood is predicted to be below 55 millimeters of mercury, then you need to have supplemental oxygen on the airplane during the flight.

Once it has been determined that you need supplemental oxygen for air travel, you can make arrangements for in-flight oxygen with the commercial carrier at least forty-eight hours before departure. If you are already on oxygen due to medical necessity under normal circumstances, similar arrangements are required.

Needless to say, continue to keep your lung function in optimal condition with consistent use of bronchodilators, expectorants, and, as indicated, corticosteroids.

Immunizations

Immunizations are so important for anyone with respiratory illness. These should receive the same priority as vaccinations with your child because vaccine-preventable deaths occur predominantly in adults.

Pneumococcal Vaccine

To avoid getting pneumonia, you might ask your doctor about the pneumococcal vaccine (Pneumovax or Pneu-Immune 23). The currently available vaccine is safe and not expensive. It provides immunity against twenty to thirty subtypes of bacteria that commonly cause pneumonia.

If you are a healthy adult over sixty-five, this vaccine is recommended. Some experts suggest that this be given at an earlier age (less than fifty-five) when the immune responsiveness is greater. It is also recommended for those at increased risk for infection, such as those with chronic medical problems such as liver or heart disease, COPD, kidney failure, diabetes, a variety of cancers, and sickle-cell anemia. If you have had your spleen removed or have had a disease that affects the function of the spleen, you should also get Pneumovax. The vaccine should not be given to a woman during pregnancy.

Influenza Vaccine

The annual influenza epidemics have caused 10,000 deaths since 1957. These occurred despite the availability of influenza vaccines. The protection provided by the vaccine is due to the production of antibodies against the virus. In young adults, immunization provides 65 to 80 percent protection against illness due to the virus which the vaccine is designed to stimulate immunity against. In the elderly, the vaccine may be only 30 to 40 percent effective in preventing illness, but it lessens the severity of the disease and prevents hospital admission and death.

The influenza vaccine, known as Fluvax, is recommended for anyone older than sixty-five, as well as health care workers and those with conditions that place them at high risk (similar to the high-risk groups mentioned for Pneumovax).

The virus changes each year so a new vaccination is required each fall. There are usually two strains of influenza A and one strain of influenza B in each year's vaccine. The vaccine is considered safe and effective. Risk-benefit studies have consistently shown that the risk of deaths from influenza outweighs the potential for adverse vaccine reactions for all age groups.

The vaccine should not be given to pregnant women or to those who are allergic to eggs. One-third of people receiving the Fluvax have a mild local reaction at the site of injection. A very few experience a low-grade fever and generalized achiness six to twelve hours after the injection, which may last one or two days. There are rare allergic reactions.

If necessary, Pneumovax and Fluvax may be given on the same day as long as each vaccine is injected from a separate syringe at different sites.

Surgery

Besides these conventional medications, those with severe emphysema might want to consider *lung volume reduction surgery* or *reduction pneumoplasty*. This procedure involves surgically removing the most-damaged areas of your lung so the remaining volume that was previously compressed will expand appropriately. This may improve your overall lung function.

Many have experienced significant improvements in lung function as well as exercise tolerance after this surgery. In addition, more than half of those who are dependent on oxygen before the procedure have been able to safely stop oxygen use afterward.

Although lung volume reduction surgery is not endorsed as a standard treatment for emphysema, the promising results suggest the need for continued study. This is ongoing at specially designated medical centers around the country. Talk with your doctor and see whether this might be a consideration for your case.

More Tools for Better Breathing

A Nebulizer System

As discussed on page 101, for those who are unable to use inhaled medications with spacers effectively, their physicians may prescribe a nebulizer system. This portable machine is similar to the device hospitals use and allows liquid medication to turn into a mist as it is inhaled into the lungs. A face mask or mouthpiece may be used, depending on the patient's ability to inhale properly.

Solutions for the nebulizer are prescribed in either a ready-to-use form or a concentrated form, which needs to be diluted. Your doctor will guide you in how to pour these solutions into the nebulizer. Once the solution has been mixed, the total time for nebulization takes between five and fifteen minutes. Nebulizers are cumbersome and more expensive than MDIs with spacers.

Mucus Clearance Device

A small handheld device called the Flutter was developed in the mid-eighties in Switzerland, and newer studies show that this may be useful for those with chronic bronchitis, asthma, or cystic fibrosis. To use the Flutter, the patient exhales into the plastic mouthpiece. A stainless steel ball, which rests in a plastic circular cone on the inside of the Flutter, begins to roll up and down as the patient breathes. This creates oscillations in the airflow from the lungs, resulting in vibrations, or a "fluttering" sensation. The oscillations are supposed to loosen the mucus from the airway walls. Some promising studies have shown that daily use of the Flutter can increase the peak flow rate of some with respiratory problems.

The Flutter has Food and Drug Administration approval for those with cystic fibrosis, bronchitis, and bronchiectasis and is available by prescription. Ask your doctor for more information about the Flutter or write to Scandipharm, Inc., 22 Inverness Center Parkway, Suite 310, Birmingham, AL 35242 (800–950–8085). You can also contact the Cystic Fibrosis Foundation, 6931 Arlington Road, Bethesda, MD 20814 (800–344–4823).

Nasal Strips

The Food and Drug Administration has approved Breathe Right Nasal Strips to help relieve congestion and nasal stuffiness. These strips of tape are placed over the bridge of the nose; then a plastic strip springs back and helps gently open your nasal passages and reduce airflow resistance. This drug-free measure for better breathing is also said to help reduce snoring to some extent in some people who wear them. Breathe Right Nasal Strips come in three sizes and are available in most pharmacies and grocery stores.

Familiarity with Your Medications

Asking questions before taking any medication is important. Some drug interactions can happen unexpectedly whereas others are quite predictable. Be sure to keep a current and accurate medication record, including both prescription and nonprescription medications that you take. A thorough understanding of each medication is necessary. For example, inhaled corticosteroids will not relieve acute bronchoconstriction but an inhaled beta2-agonist will. Getting this information confused may make you wonder why the inhaler is not opening your breathing passages and possibly place you in a precarious position.

Try to use only one pharmacy so your pharmacist can keep a record of each medication. Sometimes the pharmacist may alert the physician if a patient is using too much of one medication or not enough of another or if a dangerous drug-drug interaction could occur. Seek help and information from professionals but continue to be actively involved in the process by being aware of all medicines you are using. It is essential to know the names, doses, reasons for using, and the potential side effects of the drugs you are taking.

Immunotherapy

If you find that medications are not effective in reducing allergy and asthma symptoms, your doctor may suggest allergy shots (injections or immunotherapy). Injections or allergy shots are effective for reducing allergic symptoms associated with cat dander, pollens, house dust mites, certain molds, and fire ant bites. Regular injections of allergens, given in increasing doses, stimulate changes in the immune system that decrease the chance of future allergic reactions.

Once your physician has helped you to identify the allergens that trigger your symptoms by taking your medical history and allergy testing, a series of injections with solutions containing increasing concentrations of these allergens may be used to lessen your sensitivity and reduce symptoms. These shots, which are the only known way to turn off allergic disease, reduce the production of IgE and cause the body to make another class of antibody called "blocking-IgG." The blocking-IgG antibody helps protect you from allergic diseases. Shots are the only method available for long-lasting protection from allergies, particularly allergic rhinitis. They have been effective in a few cases of specially selected asthma patients, although new studies suggest that this may not be true.

Studies have found that 85 percent of the people who receive allergy shots to treat hay fever due to grass, ragweed, trees, and dust get better. Your doctor will give shots of weak allergen solutions once or twice a week initially and then gradually increase the strength of the solution. When you reach the strongest dosage, you may receive the injections only once a month. The results are not immediate and estimates are that it takes three to five years to reach an optimal benefit. Many people get better for years and some even permanently.

Find What Works

Take advantage of the myriad of new medical treatments. There are enough choices that most people should find something to help them breathe better. Talk about these options with your doctor and, together, decide on the treatment combination that works best for you and allows for greater activity and enjoyment of your life.

chapter 6

Avoiding Triggers

On guard! That is the motto of anyone with respiratory problems, and you know what we mean. Being on guard means always taking tissues, inhalers, nasal sprays, and other medications with you no matter where you go. It includes avoiding the out-of-doors when the pollen count is high, staying out of wind, rain and cold weather, and dodging any pollutants, smoke, or fumes like the plague, for no matter what time of year it is, some allergen or trigger is always lurking in the air just waiting to cause your next "respiratory revolution."

So, what is out there taking your breath away? A wide array of often invisible but deleterious things. Invisible particles, including dust mites, pollens, molds, and animal dander can become trapped in tightly insulated and poorly ventilated areas, whether at your home or office. These pollutants infiltrate the air you breathe and trigger coughs and nasal drainage. One revealing study found an allergen level to be 200 percent higher in a tightly insulated home as opposed to a home that is not as well insulated.

What you may have thought of as simply the culprit for a housekeeping chore—dust—is one top breath stealer because it is filled with live organisms. Dust mites may be to blame for 50 to 80 percent of all asthma cases. These insect-like creatures grow where it is warm and humid and breed rampantly in pillows, mattresses, and upholstery. They feast primarily on a diet of your skin scales, and their waste causes chronic allergic symptoms in more than 20 million Americans.

Adding to air pollution are environmental chemicals used at home and work that cause health problems such as dizziness, shortness of breath, and respiratory distress. Check the labels on your cleaning solvents. The skull and crossbones symbol is there for a reason! If you have ever sniffed drain cleaner or inhaled a soap scum remover in a nonventilated area, you already know those chemicals can wreak havoc with your airways.

The World Health Organization estimates that 20 to 30 percent of office workers around the globe suffer from some form of sick building syndrome, with more than 30 percent of new or refurbished offices at risk. Because of well-built homes, there is a good chance the air you breathe at night is sick, too.

Another environmental hazard for home or office is the threat of carbon monoxide poisoning. Carbon monoxide is a colorless, odorless gas that can be formed in natural gas, oil, or propane-fueled home heating systems and in wood-burning fireplaces, as well as gas ovens, stove tops, and charcoal grills. A low level of carbon monoxide may cause flulike symptoms; at higher levels, it causes headaches and nausea. Even higher levels can result in respiratory failure, convulsions, coma, and even death.

A carbon monoxide detector, available at hardware and home center stores for around $30 to $50, can sense an unsafe level of carbon monoxide and sound a warning. A detector should be installed close to each bedroom.

Environmental Factors

Asthma, allergy, COPD, and other respiratory disorders may be affected not only by your work environment but also by your home environment and hobby exposures and by airborne particles. It is well known that exposure to environmental allergens such as ragweeds, pollens, and grasses can exacerbate a person's allergies or asthma, particularly if they are of the IgE-dependent type. Evidence is building that exposure to cockroaches can lead susceptible people to develop asthma; this provides some explanation for the finding of more asthma among the poor and inner-city population than among the middle and upper classes.

Exposure to certain pets can make asthma worse. Pets in the cat, rodent, and ornamental bird families are particularly associated with the development and exacerbations of asthma. This is due to exposure to proteins in the skin or urine of these animals. Exposure to certain ornamental birds is also associated with a different type of lung inflammation called *hypersensitivity pneumonitis,* which has symptoms similar to those of asthma.

Similarly, hobby substances that can also lead to the development or exacerbation of asthma include acid anhydrides present in epoxy resins and paints, metal fumes and salts such as chrome, nickel, or particularly platinum. Wood workers may have asthma attacks triggered by wood dust, particularly mahogany, oak, Western red cedar, and California redwood. Flour may cause asthma in some people who do baking or handle baked goods.

Studies have found that exposure to air pollution can affect the respiratory system in various ways, including impeding the lungs' ability to function due to inflammation and destruction of lung tissue. Dangerous pollutants include the following:

Ozone

Ozone is the major destructive ingredient in smog. It causes coughing, shortness of breath, and chest pain. It also boosts the susceptibility to infection. At high concentrations, ozone can scar the lungs. People who exercise out-of-doors are particularly vulnerable to the effects of ozone.

Sulfur Dioxide

Sulfur dioxide, another component of smog, is created when sulfur-containing fuel is burned. It irritates the airways and constricts the air passages, and so causes asthma attacks. It can suppress mucousal ciliary action and can set the stage for permanent lung damage.

Nitrogen Dioxide

This is produced when fuel is burned, especially by motor vehicles and power plants. Nitrogen dioxide contributes to ozone formation. It causes bronchitis and, like ozone, increases the susceptibility to infection. One study revealed that those who cook on gas stoves may be more prone to hay fever and asthma-related symptoms, wheezing and breathlessness, because of the released nitrogen dioxide.

Carbon Monoxide

This odorless, colorless gas comes mainly from automobile and other combustion exhausts. It reduces oxygen levels in the blood, and so starves the body's cells. It is especially dangerous for people with heart disease and unborn or newborn children.

To protect yourself from air pollution, be aware of reports that tell of pollution levels' being high and avoid going out-of-doors during this time. If you must leave your home or office, avoid strenuous activity and long-term exposure.

Controlling Your Environment

No matter what the air quality in your home or workplace, it is time to become proactive for cleaner air. It is important to get rid of as many triggers as you can and then try to keep the others under control.

Go through your home or office, and discover the problem areas. Although environmental triggers vary, common triggers include:

Aerosols	Mold and mildew
Chemical fumes	Perfume and scented
Cigarette smoke	products
Cockroaches	Pet dander
Cold air	Pollen
Dust	Tobacco and wood smoke
Fresh paint	Weather fronts
Humid air	Wind

In the workplace, there is an enormous range of potential environmental substances you are exposed to that can cause respiratory distress, including animal-derived material (dander and secretions), plants and vegetable products (cotton or grain dust), wood dusts, chemicals, dyes, fumes, and salts.

Dust Mites

An estimated 500 million people around the world are allergic to dust mites. Some studies suggest that this allergen may be a factor in as many as 80 percent of all asthma cases.

Since dust is a key cause of many allergic symptoms,

studies show that decreasing your exposure can help greatly to decrease your symptoms. Scientists have recently reported that there is an obvious relationship between the level of exposure to house dust mite allergens and the severity of asthma in children. Studies of Australian children who were exposed to dust mites, a common household allergen, showed that these children were more likely to have asthma. Researchers agreed that if the allergen levels could be reduced, the severity of children's asthma might also be diminished. If you could stop asthma from being chronic in childhood, it might not be such a severe disease throughout the rest of life.

One gram of dust may contain as many as 250,000 dust mite feces. It is this waste that makes you sneeze and wheeze. The following preventive measures can help you eliminate as much of this waste as possible:

Use air conditioning during warm and hot months. This will filter the air and take out more than 99 percent of all the pollen and allergen-producing material.

Ask your heating and air-conditioning service contractor to inspect the air ducts in your home, and consider having these professionally cleaned.

Dust at least once a week or more often if possible.

Wear a dust mask when you clean, use nonporous vacuum cleaner bags, and try to find a vacuum with a High Efficiency Particulate Arrestor (HEPA) filter to help eliminate dust. A HEPA filter is efficient in filtering out almost 100 percent of airborne allergens and danders.

Eliminate dust mites by getting rid of fuzzy or woolen blankets and down comforters, and wash bed linens in hot water.

Encase your mattress and pillow in a plastic zip-on cover to prevent dust mites in your bedding. These can be purchased at any allergy supply store. Tape over the zipper to seal dust leaks.

Modify your home and work space by replacing dusty carpets with linoleum or hardwood floors and moldy curtains with shades or easy-wipe shutters.

Use a solution of 3 percent tannic acid to neutralize the allergen in dust mite droppings. Acarosan (benzyl benzoate) can be purchased at an allergy supply store. This powder is sprinkled onto carpets and vacuumed after it has dried. Acarosan will kill mites, neutralize the allergenic shedding, and make it easier to remove these allergens when vacuuming.

Keep your house cool (less than 70 degrees) and dry (less than 50 percent relative humidity; 30 to 40 percent is ideal). Both measures help decrease the abundance of dust mites, as well as cockroaches and fungal problems.

Purchase a humidity gauge to let you know when your home is too humid (more than 50 percent) as mites grow best at 70 to 80 percent humidity and cannot live in less than 50 percent humidity.

Purchase a dehumidifier to keep the indoor humidity less than 50 percent, but be sure to clean it regularly. Fans might help, too, but keep the exhaust toward the outside.

Maximize the air flow inside your home, along with reducing the dust and mold, by leaving the doors open between the rooms.

Avoid using humidifiers and vaporizers as these can increase the dust mite and mold growth. If you use these, be sure you empty and clean them daily.

Use several layers of cheesecloth as a filter over incoming air vents. These will help to trap dust, dirt, or lint coming through the duct work.

If possible, keep clothing in another room to lessen dust in the bedroom.

Launder your clothes frequently. Dust mites thrive in clothing in which perspiration provides a moist environment. A cold water wash will get rid of some dust mites, but only hot water (at least 131 degrees Fahrenheit) will kill the mites.

Purchase a HEPA room-sized air filter for your bedroom.

Cockroaches

In the past five years, asthma has increasingly become a severe urban health concern with cockroaches as the surprising trigger. Researchers have found that the more cockroaches one has in the home, the greater the chance of allergy and severity of asthma symptoms. Asthma in children is generally triggered by a reaction to a substance called an antigen. After many studies in children under age ten, the proteins in the carcasses and droppings of the German cockroach were found to be the greatest antigen and asthma trigger.

The increase of cockroaches as asthma triggers is partly because of tightly insulated newer homes where there is little air exchange. This causes a definite buildup in the home of antigens from bugs, molds, and animals. Wall-to-wall carpeting adds to the problem as it is filled with antigens. An even greater problem arises when you try to eliminate cockroaches from your home or workplace as the fumes and chemicals from pesticides can also trigger asthma. In fact, this is one of the most frequent causes of emergency room visits.

What can you do to safely decrease the cockroach problem?

Put weather stripping around your doors to eliminate unwanted guests from entering your home.

Seal holes around pipes.

Always put food away after eating or cooking.

Wipe counters to eliminate food crumbs and make sure floors are clean.

Keep garbage cans closed tightly.

If you do use an exterminator, request that the chemicals used are unscented. Make sure your family stays out of the home the day of spraying and air your house to remove any fumes.

Molds and Mildew

Mildew is caused by molds, which are parasitic, microscopic fungi without stems, roots, or leaves. Mold spores appear outside after spring and reach their peak from midsummer to October. In the South and on the West Coast, mold spores can be found year-round.

Molds are present almost anywhere. Outside, they can be found in soil, rotting wood, or vegetation, such as wet leaves or mulch, outdoor vinyl furniture, outdoor cushions, patios, and boat canvas. Inside, molds are found in bathrooms, bedrooms, refrigerators, garages, attics, garbage containers, carpets, damp wallpaper, rotting wood floors, and upholstery.

Preventing molds requires finding ways to provide good ventilation, light, dryness, and cleanliness for your home. Consider the following important measures as you work to impede the growth of mold:

Change your home or office air filter at least every other month, or consider changing to a HEPA air filter to improve air quality.

Keep your kitchen and bathroom surfaces dry. Use diluted bleach, if necessary, to remove any mildew in musty areas.

Fix any leaky pipes or cracks and crevices to avoid water leakage in the home.

Get rid of indoor plants and other sources of mildew.

Purchase an ultraviolet light that will eliminate mold spores if it is on. These are used in hospitals to kill bacteria and viruses, but mold spores are also sensitive to this wavelength.

Try Silica-Gel (available under different trade names) to stop mold growth by absorbing moisture from the air. This is a mixture of activated alumina and calcium chloride.

Animals

Most pets can cause allergies, especially cats and dogs. Although cats usually produce more severe allergic reactions than dogs, both species affect approximately 15 percent of the population and 20 to 30 percent of those with asthma. Some recent studies have suggested that male cats are more likely to make you sneeze. Fur and skin tests showed that female cats produced one-third fewer allergy-causing proteins (allergens) than the males. The production of cat allergen is thought to be triggered by the predominantly male hormone testosterone.

You may be allergic to a protein found in the saliva, dander, or urine of the animal. When the animal grooms, this allergen is carried through the air on invisible particles and then lands on the lining of your eyes and nose. It may be inhaled directly into the lungs. Pet allergies can also affect the skin and cause hives and itching. The animal's hair or fur can collect dust, pollen, mold, or other allergens and bring them into the home.

Bird droppings are another source of dust, fungi, mold, and bacteria. The droppings of other caged pets, such as hamsters or gerbils, also breed these allergens.

Try the following important prevention measures if you have a pet.

Keep your pet outside your home. If you find this difficult, at least keep it out of your bedroom. Even if you do remove the pet, it can take weeks to months before the pet allergen is all gone.

Keep all animals clean, and wash them weekly in lukewarm water without soap. Studies show that this may reduce the amount of dander and dried saliva deposited on furniture and elsewhere.

Let nonallergic family members or friends bathe the animal and clean the bedding, litter box, or cage.

Find a new home for that beloved pet if your symptoms are chronic, or trade it for tropical fish.

Pollen

Allergic rhinitis is primarily caused by pollens and affects more than 15 percent of all Americans. These microscopic powdery granules of flowering plants are the mechanisms for the fertilization of trees, grasses, and weeds. Every plant has a specific period of pollination. Although weather changes can determine the pollen count in the air, the pollinating season stays constant. It can begin in January in the South; however, generally plants pollinate from early spring until October.

Pollen is a never-ending story with trees' pollinating first during springtime, grasses' pollinating from late spring to midsummer, and weeds' pollinating in late summer and early fall. When the weather is cloudy or rainy, pollen does not move about, although some botanists have discovered an allergen inside grass pollen released into the air when the pollen is ruptured by water.

Allergy and asthma sufferers must cautiously watch those dry, hot, or windy days when pollen is heavily distributed. In fact, because pollen travels for many miles, many different trees, grasses, and weeds can cause you problems, not just the ones in your yard.

Some researchers have found an association between pollen allergies and food allergies. There is evidence that a family of proteins called profilins, which are present in many plant species, are capable of acting as panallergens. Profilin sensitization from birch tree pollen and other pollens has been shown to cross-react with sensitization to many fresh fruits and vegetables.

During times of heavy pollen, it is important to follow a few rules for easier breathing:

Stay indoors and keep your windows closed, especially during heavy pollen times.

Shower, wash hair, and change clothing after being out-of-doors.

Use air conditioning that cleans, cools, and dries the air.

Keep car windows closed to avoid pollen during travel.

Purchase a portable HEPA air filter for your bedroom (around $300). Air filters clean the air that passes through the filtration system.

Consider immunotherapy to reduce hypersensitivity (see pages 116–17).

Hire someone to take care of your lawn during peak pollen season.

Wear glasses or sunglasses outdoors to protect your eyes from airborne pollen.

Avoid outdoor activities during peak pollen and mold time—between 5 and 10 A.M.

If pollen is a main trigger for your breathing problems, you are probably allergic to oak, maple, poplar, sweetgum, sycamore, and pecan trees, as well as Bermuda grass and ragweed. Showier plants that are pollinated by insects can be less bothersome for those with allergy or asthma. These plants have larger pollen grains, which are less likely to be inhaled. The American Lung Association recommends that you use the following "sneezeless" plants in your landscape:

TREES Dogwood, pear, pine, redbud, tulip, crepe myrtle, palm, and magnolia
SHRUBS Boxwood, pyracantha, and hibiscus
FLOWERS Azalea, begonia, bougainvillea, camellia, poppy, iris, tulip, and pansy

Be aware of the pollen count, which is usually shown during weather reports or on the Aeroallergen Network. The level of pollen could be classified as absent, low, moderate, high, or very high. (Even though the pollen count may be classified as low, airborne pollen out-of-doors can still cause allergy or asthma problems. The best advice is to play it safe. Always premedicate and take reliever medications with you in case of breathing emergencies, no matter what the pollen count.)

Smoke and Gas

Heating and cooking with gas could be potentially harmful to those with respiratory problems. British researchers found that women who cooked with gas were more likely to have had wheezing, breathlessness, asthma attacks, and hay fever during the year than women who cooked with other methods. Nitrogen dioxide, a product of gas heating, may be the culprit.

Being around any type of smoke is a problem for those with breathing problems. Although smoke is not an allergen, it can definitely irritate sensitive airways. Avoid being around cigarette smoke or smoke from an indoor fireplace, wood-burning stove or heater, or outdoor barbeque grill.

Use the following preventive measures to avoid smoke and gas:

If you cook on a gas stove, consider purchasing an electric unit. If you cannot do this, consider having ceiling fans installed in your kitchen for better air circulation.

Convert gas heat to electric heat in your home.

Convert wood-burning stoves or fireplaces to electric.

Designate a "smokers" area in your home such as the back porch.

Make sure your work station is away from smokers.

Leave rooms where people are smoking cigarettes, and ask for meetings to be held in a well-ventilated room.

Always choose the no smoking section of restaurants and public dwellings.

Purchase a HEPA filter to help absorb smoke and chemical gases.

Have coworkers agree to leave the room when they smoke.

All Air Filters Are Not Created Equal

REGULAR AIR CONDITIONING AND HEATING FILTERS

are effective in removing particles down to about 10 microns, and central systems are more effective than window units. Most mold spores and fine dust continue to circulate as they are too small to be removed.

ELECTROSTATIC FILTERS

remove particles (down to 0.01 micron in size) by static electricity and create an electrostatic charge as air passes through the special filter material, which causes it to attract and hold contaminant particles.

HEPA (HIGH EFFICIENCY PARTICULATE ARRESTOR) FILTERS

are efficient in filtering almost 100 percent of airborne dander and allergens. Some vacuum cleaners are equipped with HEPA filters. Small units that can filter all the air in a 9- by 12-foot room six times in one hour can be purchased for about $100.

NEGATIVE ION GENERATORS

are less standardized than the other three. They produce negative ions to increase the healthful balance of ions in a home and also precipitate dust and mold particles on the curtains and walls.

Chemicals

More than a half-million Americans have asthma caused by inhaling chemicals or other types of irritants at work. The most common asthma-causing chemicals are *isocyanates*. These chemicals are used to make foam for chairs and car seats and are found in glue and spray paint. Other hazardous workplace chemicals are proteolytic enzymes—components of detergent.

To avoid problems from chemicals, take the following measures:

Make sure your home or office has good ventilation.

Purchase new equipment as improved equipment design can reduce the production of vapors, mists, and splashes. Enclose the equipment to keep any fumes from polluting the air.

Replace or recover furniture as some fabrics give off chemical smells, especially formaldehyde, which can irritate the eyes, nose, and breathing passages.

Keep your home well-ventilated for at least forty-eight hours after the installation of new carpeting. Potentially harmful volatile organic compounds (VOCs) are released into the air from new carpets.

Avoid household products (cleaning agents, pesticides, and paints) that are dangerous or may trigger respiratory problems.

Avoid aerosol sprays, perfumes, talcum powder, room deodorizers, nail polish and remover, and other sources of strong odors.

Weather Conditions

There are many weather conditions that trigger respiratory problems, including dry air, cold air, humidity, fronts, and wind. Exposure to cold air causes several effects on the respiratory system such as airway congestion, bronchoconstriction, secretions, and decreased mucociliary clearance.

Interestingly, an asthma epidemic occurred in London in June 1994 immediately following a thunderstorm. This resulted in more than 640 patients' being treated for asthma or other airway diseases during thirty hours— nearly ten times the expected number. New episodes of asthma were significantly associated with a drop in air temperature six hours previously and a high grass pollen concentration nine hours previously. While first-time episodes of asthma during the epidemic on June 24 and

25 were associated with a fall in air temperature and a rise in grass pollen concentration, nonepidemic asthma was significantly associated with other environmental stimuli, including the following triggers:

Lightning strikes
Increase in humidity
Increase in sulfur dioxide concentration
Drop in temperature the previous day
High rainfall the previous day
Decrease in the maximum air pressure
Changes in grass pollen counts over the previous two days

You can avoid weather-related allergies or asthma by staying out of cold air, wind, rain, and other conditions that trigger your symptoms.

Avoidance Is Crucial

Avoidance is vital for controlling the symptoms triggered by environmental factors. Steps such as staying away from cleaning chemicals, avoiding touching the cat or dog, and going into another room if someone is smoking should become habitual behavioral responses. If your workplace is full of fumes or chemicals that trigger respiratory distress, ask your employer to move you to another office or consider changing jobs.

Remember, no one can do it for you. Once you understand your disease, as well as the specific allergens and triggers that cause symptoms in your respiratory system, it is crucial to use the proactive steps recommended for better breathing.

chapter 7

Achieving Optimal Fitness

Until recently, many doctors felt that exercise might exacerate the symptoms of chronic respiratory diseases; thus they encouraged patients to seek rest, not activity. Three decades ago, children who suffered from asthma, bronchitis, or allergy stood passively on the sidelines instead of competing in the race. However, in the past two decades, researchers have become increasingly aware of the importance of conditioning exercise and activity for optimum respiratory function.

There is a growing body of evidence that links exercise with better breathing and improved management of respiratory problems. Recent studies show that people with breathing disorders who can maintain a regular program of exercise and activity are able to experience maximum cardiovascular fitness along with greater symptom control, or an increased ability to exercise and do the activities of daily living. Exercise trains the respiratory muscles to work more efficiently.

An excellent example of the benefit of exercise—and the detriment of its absence—is COPD. Many people with this disease think they cannot exercise, so they quit moving around altogether. This lack of aerobic fitness leaves the person out of shape, out of breath, and unable to function in her daily routine because she is aerobically unfit. On the other hand, when someone with COPD starts doing moderate exercise (with her physician's approval and proper medication), she will find that her endurance and cardiovascular function both improve; this helps increase her activity and quality of life.

"But I have chronic lung disease," you may say. "I would be active if my lungs were functioning better." It is important to understand lung function when you live with breathing disorders. As you will learn in this chapter, exercise and activity are the keys to better breathing and optimal health. For healthy individuals and for those with breathing problems, exercise and activity work the same. They recondition your breathing muscles so you can take deeper breaths, and boost the oxygen level in the blood.

An excellent example of aerobically fit individuals with lung disease who are managing symptoms with exercise are the Olympic athletes. In the 1984 and 1988 Olympics, approximately 120 athletes with asthma competed and 57 of them won medals! Olympic decathlete Rob Muzzio tells of his personal battle with asthma in the Foreword of this book. Jackie Joyner-Kersee, Nancy Hogshead, Jim Ryun, Amy Van Dyken, and Tom Dolan all have asthma, and all were Olympic medalists. These athletes learned quickly that with proper medication and exercise, managing breathing disorders is possible, and they could fulfill their dreams.

The Active Way to Better Breathing

A great deal of literature exists on the beneficial effects of exercise training in people who do *not* have respiratory problems; the principles remain the same for people with breathing problems. Clearly, if you have breathing problems, they limit your ability to move air in and out of your lungs. If you cannot persuade your lungs to move any more air in and out, then you need to be able to do more with the air you can move.

When it comes to exertion and exercise, many who suffer with breathing disorders have extremely inadequate levels of physical fitness. A problem arises because exercise and activity demand more oxygen—the very thing they may not have. When you hyperventilate with vigorous exercise, the airway may be cooled; this causes the release of *leukotrienes,* which can trigger wheezing due to the constriction of bronchial tubes in those who are susceptible. Those who live with the headache of chronic sinusitis have a difficult time just getting through the day, much less exercising. For sufferers of allergic rhinitis, trying to run, play soccer, or even swim with a congested nose is close to impossible.

So, what is the answer? Do you exercise and risk having an allergy, asthma, or wheezing attack or not? The answer may surprise you.

It is a known fact that if you exercise vigorously on a regular basis, then you should become more aerobically fit. In other words, you can do the same amount of work with less oxygen. This means that if your body was rated as a machine, then you would now be more efficient. This fact is well accepted for people who do not have breathing problems, but it is also true for those with breathing disorders. To understand the principle better, you might use the analogy of a motor vehicle engine.

Consider your heart as the fuel pump and the muscles of the arms and legs as the motor. Obviously, the bigger the pump, the more fuel it can send to the motor, and the more power the motor can produce. Similarly, the bigger the heart muscles, the more fuel it can send to the muscles if the heart is not diseased. The bigger the muscles of your arms and legs, the more power you can produce when everything else is working at its best.

This analogy works well for the air intake of a car. For a car to be able to burn fuel, it must have oxygen from the air. The greater the air intake, the more oxygen it can consume in a given amount of time. This is analogous to the amount of air you can breathe while exercising. Obviously, if you have a restricted air intake, then the maximum amount of power you can produce is restricted.

Your car engine performs work. The maximum amount of work it can perform in a certain amount of time determines its *power rating*. In automotive terms, this is the number of *horsepower*. For automobiles, to build an engine with more horsepower, you have to build a bigger engine. Interestingly, human beings are in a far superior situation than a mechanic when it comes to increasing available power. The automobile mechanic cannot increase the size of your car motor without doing some serious reengineering. On the other hand, you can increase the size of any of your muscles simply through exercise. You increase not only the size of the muscles that are specifically exercised but also the size of your heart. Study after study shows that if you exercise enough, your heart muscle gets thicker and stronger. This allows it to contract with more force each time it pumps; that is, your internal "fuel pump" can operate at a higher pressure.

When exercise occurs, the amount of blood pumped with each stroke, or heart beat, increases. Consequently, if you continue to exercise regularly, your heart does not need to beat as fast to pump the same amount of blood. (If this were true for cars, the more you drove them and the faster you went, the bigger your fuel pump and engine would get!)

This analogy also works well for the power-to-weight ratio, the amount of power available per pound of engine weight. For our purposes, it is more helpful to consider the amount of power available per pound of overall car weight, including everything in it. In other words, for an engine of a particular power rating, the performance of the vehicle is better the *less* the whole car weighs. As far as a car is concerned, your only options would be to remove those few hundred pounds of junk from the trunk or heave out any spare tires.

The good news is that when you exercise, you do not have to run the risk of losing a few of your friends. Instead, you have the opportunity of gaining some. As you exercise on a regular basis, you not only lose some fat but also gain some muscle. This means that as you change "dead weight" into additional power, you improve your power-to-weight ratio and become more efficient.

Unfortunately, the more weight you carry around, the more oxygen you need to perform any particular task. This makes your heart and lungs work harder and means that as a machine is rated, you are now rated less efficient. As a simple experiment, you might try to carry a 1-gallon milk jug up and down a flight of stairs a couple of times; then try the same thing without the extra weight. The jug weighs approximately 8 pounds when full, and you can easily appreciate how much extra effort those few pounds require.

If you are in the process of trying to lose a few pounds, repeat this experiment every time you have a yearning to overeat. That way you will not only reinforce your determination to lose weight, but you may help to speed up the process.

Aerobic Benefit

The human body has two main ways of producing energy from fuel. The more efficient way is called aerobic. This is analogous to burning your gasoline completely so that all the carbon in the fuel is converted to carbon dioxide. This would produce the most amount of energy per gallon of gasoline. The less efficient way is called anaerobic, which literally means without oxygen. This occurs when the demand for energy is so great that the muscles cannot use oxygen fast enough to provide energy at the required rate. To provide the additional energy, the muscles resort to the anaerobic form of energy production. This would be similar to burning your fuel in such a way that a large amount of smoke (carbon) is produced. This carbon could have produced additional energy had it been turned into carbon dioxide or carbon monoxide.

However, the body does not produce carbon as a waste product. Instead, it produces lactic acid. This acid has to be eliminated, and for that to occur, the body has to use more oxygen. It is this need for additional oxygen after the production of lactic acid that produces the situation termed "oxygen debt." And it is the need to repay this debt that leaves you panting away after your exercise is over.

The amazing thing about humans is that as they continue to exercise on a regular basis, certain changes take place in their muscles that enable them to exercise at a greater rate without having to resort to the anaerobic form of fuel consumption. This is possible because like an engine, the human muscles can be made more efficient by modifications that improve the rate at which fuel and oxygen can enter the cylinders.

For car engines, this means more intake valves to improve the rate at which fuel and oxygen can enter and more exhaust valves to improve the rate at which exhaust gases can leave. In muscles, the inflow and outflow capabilities are determined by the number of capillaries that supply that muscle. These capillaries are the small blood vessels that bring oxygen and fuel to the muscle fibers and carry away the waste products. They are analogous to the intake and exhaust manifolds on a car engine. With exercise there is an increase in the number of capillaries.

There are more benefits from exercise. *Mitochondria,* the power houses of the cell, are inside the muscle fibers. As discussed in Chapter 1, these contain the chemicals that convert fuel and oxygen to energy. Exercise produces an increase in the size and number of these mitochondria. For a particular blood flow to a muscle, more energy can be produced by more efficiently converting fuel to energy. In other words, your muscles can produce more energy by burning the fuel more completely. Like your car engine, they can produce more power with less carbon. As a part of this process, the muscles extract oxygen more completely from the blood that goes through the capillaries. This means that you can produce more power with fewer breaths, and it is this ability that makes you more aerobically fit.

Enhanced Emotional State

Not only is exercise a key factor in aerobic fitness, it is also important for revitalizing the neurochemical balance of the body that affects our emotional state. Research has shown that regular participation in aerobic training has been reported to reduce the symptoms of moderate depression and enhance psychological fitness. Exercise can even produce changes in certain chemical levels in the body, which can have an effect on the psychological state.

Endorphins are hormones in the brain associated with a happy, positive feeling. A low level of endorphins is associated with depression. During exercise, plasma levels of this substance increase and may help to alleviate the symptoms of depression. A recent *National Health and Nutrition Examination Survey* found that physically active people were half as likely to be depressed a decade later as those who were inactive.

Interestingly, there might not be a definite link between exercise intensity and mood. In fact, new evidence shows that even regular exercisers who are not in shape and do a light or moderate workout receive the same long-term stress reduction as those who are aerobically fit. This is good news for those who have avoided moving around because of the fear of shortness of breath.

Research also shows that exercise gives a protective effect for both coronary and total mortality until at least age eighty. For many diseases, exercise is a prescription for treatment that the patient can do at no monetary cost.

The healing benefits that occur to the muscles of the arms or legs when exercised occur to only those muscles and not to any others. In other words, the best benefits occur by exercising both arm and leg muscles and also abdominal and back muscles. Yet herein lies a problem if you have severe lung disease. You may not be able to exercise all these muscles at once because you just can't breathe enough to do so. The solution is to exercise your arm and leg muscles in turn, or your leg muscles one day and your arm muscles the next.

Interestingly, some research shows that people with chronic lung disease obtain more benefit from exercising their arms than their legs. This is because the arms are typically less aerobically fit to begin with and, therefore, reach their anaerobic threshold sooner than the legs do. The *anaerobic threshold* is the point at which lactic acid is produced and is the same point at which oxygen debt starts. It appears that these factors act as the stimulus for the body to produce the modifications to the muscles that were described earlier. It is as if the body responds by modifying the muscles to do a better job after it has become apparent that they are not doing a good enough job as they are. The other reason that exercising the arms may be specifically better is that some muscles that attach the arms and shoulders to the chest also help with the process of respiration. This means that as you exercise your arms, you also exercise some of the muscles that help you breathe.

Chairobics is one particular program used by respiratory therapists for those who are breathing impaired and can be performed even by those who are bedridden. Patients who have been afraid to exercise for fear of dyspnea, or shortness of breath, are led in a series of upper body exercises while sitting. Studies show that patients who participate in this type conditioning exercise report less anxiety and greater improvement in walking distance, endurance, and upper extremity strength.

Immune System Boost

Regular exercise appears to have the advantage of jump-starting the immune system, as will be discussed in Chapter 10, and thus help reduce the number of colds and flu. One reason for this may be the increase in activity of *lymphocytes,* called *killer cells,* from regular exercise, and also the increase in immunoglobulin found in the blood.

Watch your workouts, though. A study reported in *Thorax* revealed that when workouts become stressful or excessive, the body produces increased amounts of cortisol, which can inhibit the ability of certain immune cells to work properly. In fact, some research has found that endurance athletes are at increased risk for upper respiratory tract infections during periods of prolonged training, especially the one- to nine-hour period following heavy training or exercise such as marathons.

The Cycle of Inactivity

Patients frequently ask how exercise can improve mobility and decrease serious episodes of dyspnea. In fact, many are afraid to move around more for fear it will worsen their condition, especially when they experience uncomfortable shortness of breath during activity.

Shortness of breath is a symptom of many respiratory problems. For many with asthma or COPD, this inability to breathe deeply or comfortably is only worsened with exercise or activity. But vigorous exercise also causes shortness of breath for people *without* lung problems. With ongoing conditioning, this symptom improves over time.

The problem arises when those with lung disease exercise and experience shortness of breath at minimal levels of exertion. These patients may experience a cycle of inactivity that begins with increased shortness of breath and then leads to inactivity, poor physical conditioning, and finally to fatigue and even more shortness of breath on exertion. Being inactive increases the inefficiency of your muscles, so that simple tasks are almost impossible. Muscles deteriorate, or atrophy, if not used. This loss of the ability to exercise results in more inactivity—a vicious cycle.

Most patients with respiratory problems have a reduced quality of life, which can be directly related to the result of chronic symptoms that impede activity, such as shortness of breath. However, exercise and increased mobility are important components of a management plan to reduce the frequency of difficulty in breathing, improve endurance for daily activities and cardiovascular fitness, and cope with life's stressors, including the disease, in a more accepting manner. In other words, the more conditioned you become, the more you can handle activity and the better quality of life you can have.

Some patients will benefit from participation in a comprehensive pulmonary rehabilitation program, such as those offered at many hospitals around the country. These programs include education regarding the disease, its management with medication, and the importance of proper nutrition and normal weight and psychological intervention such as patient discussion groups. The most important component of the programs involves exercise, including walking as well as specific exercise to recondition the respiratory muscles by using a device called an *inspiratory muscle trainer.* This small, handheld device is put to your lips like an inhaler; then you breathe in and out through the mouthpiece. As you breathe, you will feel some resistance, which can be adjusted according to the strength of your inspiratory muscles. This resistance helps to exercise your inspiratory muscles. When you first begin using it, you want little resistance. As your muscles become stronger and your breathing improves, you can gradually increase the resistance during inspiration.

Exercise-Induced Asthma (EIA)

Exercise triggers asthma symptoms in more than 90 percent of people, children and adults, with asthma. In fact, EIA is a chronic condition affecting more than 12 percent of the country's total population, according to the American Lung Association. For most sufferers, the symptoms of coughing, wheezing, shortness of breath, or chest tightness occur after stopping exercise. Poor conditioning may be part of the cause of EIA.

Even those who have no history of asthma can be affected by EIA. Air pollution, a history of viral infections, and allergies can all contribute to this problem, which is caused by the loss of water and heat from the lungs.

Exercising in cold air can be potentially dangerous for some people. As the cold air enters the bronchial tubes, it triggers a reaction in which the muscles in the tubes constrict and mucus production is increased. The narrowing of the airway combined with the buildup of mucus causes exercise-induced asthma to occur. In the Winter Olympics in Lillehammer, Norway, 24 percent of the Nordic ski competitors were found to have asthma.

Difficulty breathing during and after activity can discourage a person to exercise. However, after starting a

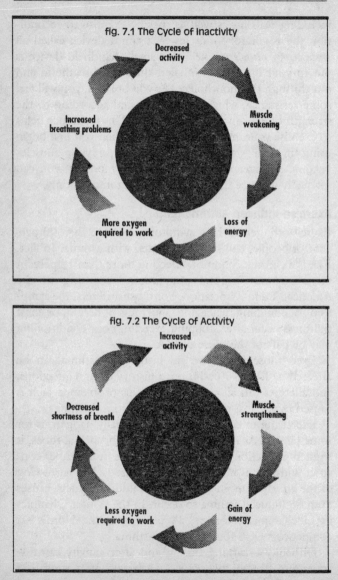

fig. 7.1 The Cycle of Inactivity

Decreased activity

Muscle weakening

Loss of energy

More oxygen required to work

Increased breathing problems

fig. 7.2 The Cycle of Activity

Increased activity

Muscle strengthening

Gain of energy

Less oxygen required to work

Decreased shortness of breath

conditioning program and with pretreatment, many people with exercise-induced asthma will benefit from lower resting and maximum heart rates because of the increased aerobic activity. Participation in their sport of choice should be the goal of all EIA patients.

Pretreatment Is Necessary

Pretreatment is a vital part of your management plan as you begin a regular exercise program. Studies show that in about 95 percent of all cases of exercise-induced asthma, taking the proper medications (both oral and inhaled) before exercise gives adequate protection. These medications may include cromolyn sodium (Intal), nedocromil sodium (Tilade), or inhaled short-acting bronchodilator medications such as albuterol (Proventil, Ventolin).

It is also important to check your peak flow measurement before exercise. This number should give an accurate indication of your breathing function, and so let you know whether there is impairment even before you feel shortness of breath. If your peak flow rate is in a warning zone, it is important to treat your breathing problem correctly before any activity.

Practice Breathing

It appears that there is no way to avoid shortness of breath as you try to maintain aerobic fitness. It also appears, however, that merely being short of breath during exercise is not bad for you and, as has already been discussed, it is good for you in the long run. Remember to check with your physician for your special concerns.

There are three keys to proper breathing during exercise, and each of these techniques can be practiced for a period of time each day before exercise. Doing so will allow you to continue using proper breathing when you begin your walk, swim, or other exercise and give your body the ultimate benefit of oxygen.

1. Nose Breathing

When you breathe through your nose, the air becomes warm and moist before going into your airways. This breathing method is especially important as cold, dry air is a major problem and can trigger an asthma attack. A recent study reported that mouth breathing during outdoor exercise also significantly increases the ozone your lungs absorb. Ozone is one of the most dangerous air pollutants because it directly damages lung tissue. This damage can be reduced through nose breathing.

Practice nose breathing throughout the day. If you find this impossible because of nasal congestion, talk with your doctor about medication or inhalers that can help relieve the congestion.

2. Diaphragmatic Breathing

When lungs are injured by chronic disease, they lose their elasticity. This makes it difficult, if not impossible, to deflate, or push trapped stale air out. Because of the trapped air, the air sacs bulge and press down on the diaphragm; this adds to your dyspnea, or shortness of breath. People who have this problem usually rely heavily on their upper chest muscles; this makes for very inefficient breathing. Taking slow, deep abdominal breaths not only oxygenates the brain but also enables the bodily functions of heart rate and blood pressure to return to normal.

For a period of time each day, lie on the floor or a bed while resting one hand on your abdomen and one hand on your chest. Breathe in and out to the count of five and watch the hand on your stomach. If it is moving upward as you inhale, you are breathing properly.

Practice this deep diaphragmatic breathing until it

becomes second nature to you. This breathing, combined with nose and pursed lip breathing, will enable you to get through your daily exercise routine without the panic of shortness of breath.

3. Pursed Lip Breathing

Studies have found that most people with respiratory problems can exercise if they practice pursed lip breathing both before and during exercise. This involves breathing air in through the nose to warm the cold, dry air and then breathing out through pursed lips. Be sure to keep your chest and shoulders relaxed and breathe from your abdomen. The exhalation should take longer than the inhalation.

Doing pursed lip breathing will prolong your expiration and create a sensation of resistance. This type breathing causes changes in pressure in the respiratory tract which lessen the bronchoconstrictor response to exercise.

Practice the three proper breathing techniques several times a day. When you find that the stressors of your day are getting to you, stop before you have a physical reaction and breathe slowly—in and out—ten times using pursed lip breathing. This will help you to stay relaxed during times of tension and will help control the stress reaction that can trigger wheezes, shortness of breath, or cough.

Increase Exercise Slowly

There is a tremendous amount of literature about how much to exercise; the consensus is to exercise as much as you can. The good news is that the more intense the exercise per session, the longer you exercise per session, and the more frequently you exercise, the *faster* you will become aerobically fit. Even better news is that if you are aerobically unfit to begin with, you will see some improvement quickly, although it will take you more sessions to reach your maximum fitness.

Now that was the good news. The bad news is that if you stop exercising, you will revert to your previously unfit state. And it only takes between ten to sixty days to revert all the way back, depending on how much you had progressed in the first place. People who have been confined to bed for long periods during any serious illness have to start their exercise program over to redevelop their aerobic fitness.

To become more active, most people can start exercise programs by taking small steps. For example, if you have difficulty during exercise or even fear exercise because of shortness of breath, begin by walking indoors from room to room for several minutes. Try to do this several times a day; then do this once each waking hour. As you progress in strength, walk around your house or apartment; again, do this several times a day. Then, walk around your front lawn and progress to walking your neighborhood block. Your pace will depend on your fitness capability and breathing ability, but by starting small and building, most people can achieve an adequate level of fitness. Remember, exercising some is better than not at all.

Once you start your exercise program, you will find that it does not take much to make a difference in your well-being. In fact, working up to a level of thirty minutes, four to five times per week, can give a real boost to your quality of life. As your exercise routine becomes regular, you will notice a decrease in shortness of breath and an increase in endurance and muscle strength and feel uplifted in spirit.

Set Specific Goals

Goals are vital for success in anything we do. With an exercise program, setting goals will help turn your initial enthusiasm into a reality. But without specific goals, you have no way to measure growth.

Make sure that the goals you set are specific, and write them down so you will visualize the commitment. Also, make sure that the goals are realistic so you attempt something you can achieve. Review these goals frequently and make changes as necessary. Some regular exercisers find it is helpful to exercise at the same time each day and plan for this in their daily schedule.

Be sure to establish goals with your doctor that are *reasonable* for your age, physical condition, and respiratory problems. If your cardiovascular fitness is low and you suffer a great deal from shortness of breath and wheezing, go slowly. Listen to your body and stop exercising when your body tells you it is time to quit.

Start with a Warm-up

Warming up for at least fifteen minutes prior to exercise is especially important for those with respiratory problems and exercise-induced asthma. This should include walking in place for several minutes along with body stretches. This warm-up allows your heart and respiratory rate to increase gradually. Some studies have found that a fifteen-minute warm-up may even help chase away exercise-induced asthma as it can reduce the chemicals in the body that cause the constriction of the bronchi.

Personalize Your Program

Pulsed exercises, or miniworkouts, are suggested to stay fit when you have breathing disorders and diminished lung function. These ten-minute miniworkouts can be done throughout the day and can provide aerobic fitness, while allowing you to have adequate rest as you build endurance and tolerance for exercise. Pulsed exercises allow a start-stop motion, rather than continuous and vigorous exercise. An example of pulsed exercise would be playing tennis, baseball, or swimming because they allow you to have a short burst of energy along with a period of rest. In fact, swimming is the preferred exercise for those with respiratory problems because it takes place in an environment of warm, moist air. On the other hand, running is the least preferred for those with breathing problems.

The following exercises and activities can be incorporated in most management plans if they do not make it even more difficult to breathe. Only you and your doctor can determine this. Using the information given, you can evaluate which exercises or activities will be beneficial to your specific respiratory problem and which will be detrimental.

If you are considering undertaking any of the exercises described in this book, it is important to first consult with your physician to determine the type and intensity of the exercise or activity. Follow your doctor's instructions prior to exercise, and take any prescribed medications, including reliever and controller inhalers, to ward off potentially life-threatening problems. Then, incorporate the exercises and activities that you enjoy and will keep doing into your daily routine. Your goal is for the exercise to benefit your cardiovascular system *and* still be enjoyable to you.

Biking

Abdominal conditioning is vital to improving the movement of the lungs. This can be done by strengthening the diaphragm and rib muscles. While crunches may be helpful, biking and other aerobic activities are even better.

Biking is something that can be done indoors or out. For those who have a difficult time exercising out-of-doors, there are many types of stationary bikes that give you resistance, keep tally of the calories you burn and the miles you go, and are even on ground level (recumbent bikes) for those who have difficulty climbing up on a bike.

Dancing

Depending on your breathing problem, dancing can give the benefits of exercise, while strengthening the body. One study reported that in a typical night of square dancing, the dancers covered more than 5 miles. The benefit to those with respiratory problems is that they can always sit out a few dances to catch their breath.

Golf

Golf is an excellent exercise if you have shortness of breath or difficulty doing more demanding conditioning exercise. The bending and swinging motions you do while playing golf will help strengthen your upper body—important for those with asthma and COPD. If you cannot walk the course, use a golf cart and try to walk some when you go to hit the ball. You can use this game for enjoyment and for building strength in your body while getting a conditioning workout.

If you are allergic to pollen and molds, be sure you medicate before playing golf and always take emergency medications with you.

Low-Impact Aerobics

Aerobic exercise causes your heart to pump oxygen to your system. This type of exercise strengthens the heart and makes it more efficient. Be sure to ask your physician for a recommendation of the intensity of exercise that you can tolerate. Your physician or a physical therapist can also explain how to monitor your heart rate during any aerobic exercise.

Caution: If you feel short of breath during low-impact

aerobics, sit out until you recover. Remember to premedicate and always keep medications with you.

Strength Training

Strength training is an anaerobic exercise because of the constant start-stop motions. This type exercise is also excellent for building the upper body.

With strength training, not only will you get increased strength and improved muscle tone, but the emphasis on reaching and other upper-torso movements will help strengthen and stretch the diaphragm. Remember to exhale (not hold your breath) during exertion and inhale during recovery. Many people forget to do this proper breathing and risk stressing the heart muscle.

Consider consulting an exercise physiologist about your particular problem, and find a strength training program that can be incorporated into your exercise regime *without fear of injury*. With help, you can make an exercise program for your own needs, which can be done at an exercise facility or at home.

Swimming

Although there is no perfect exercise for those with respiratory problems, swimming is perhaps the best because it is performed in a humid and warm environment. Not only does swimming improve muscle tone; it helps develop lung capacity.

Most people think of swimming freestyle or other strokes when you mention aquatics, but there are a host of other movements you can do that provide aerobic benefits, yet are "kinder and gentler" for those who are out of shape. Water serves as a natural resistance load as you push against it with your arms, hips, shoulders, and thighs.

Most YMCA programs in large cities offer aquatic classes, teaching you the aerobic exercises that are helpful for those with lung disease. Trained instructors can assist you in designing a water exercise program for your specific needs.

Caution: Watch jumping into cold water, which can trigger an asthma attack in some susceptible people. If you are sensitive to chemicals, you may want to avoid chlorinated pools and find a saltwater pool.

Tennis

Playing tennis and pounding the pavement while swinging for that ball is an excellent way to stay in cardiovascular shape. However, tennis is still considered a start-stop, or pulsed, exercise.

If you have joint problems with your knees, ankles, hips, or spine, then you might want to avoid this sport. If not, an active set of tennis might be the answer for you to build endurance while strengthening your fitness level. Be sure to warm up for at least fifteen minutes to avoid EIA. You may walk around the court, use the tennis racket to help with body stretches, and practice pursed lip breathing.

Rowing

For those who have access to a canoe, shell, or indoor hydraulic cylinder rower, rowing is a great aerobic exercise and can strengthen and stretch the upper body. Even the leg muscles are strengthened as you put weight on these when pulling the oars with your arms.

Rowing can be especially straining on the heart and lungs. See your physician before embarking on this sport, and start slowly.

Walking

Walking is an exercise that can be done by everyone, any time and any place. This low-impact form of exercise is less likely to cause an injury than running or low-impact aerobics and provides the added benefit of cardiovascular fitness.

If allergies trigger breathing problems, you should try to filter the incoming air during exercise by using a surgical mask or scarf. Exercising near water may also help as when airborne pollen falls into the water, it stays there.

For those with allergies who do not want to walk out-of-doors, mall walking has become popular everywhere. This allows you to benefit from exercise yet stay protected from inclement weather, pollen, air pollution, or other asthma triggers. Electronic treadmills are another solution, allowing you to continue to exercise any time of day or night. Similarly, simulated cross-country skiing as on equipment such as NordicTrack can be a good idea for those who wish to increase strength and endurance in upper and lower extremities at the same time.

Finish with a Cooldown

A fifteen-minute cooldown after your workout allows your heart rate to decrease gradually and helps to prevent muscle soreness. Use activities such as walking at a slower pace, stretching, or riding a stationary bicycle to cool down.

If you become increasingly short of breath, dizzy, or nauseated or have palpitations or chest pain during exercise, stop the activity immediately and consult your physician.

Checking Your Pulse

It is important to stay within a heart rate zone during exercise to avoid putting too much stress on the heart. Check with your physician to see what your heart rate zone should be.

To check your target heart rate zone, take your pulse

periodically. You can find a pulse by placing your finger (not your thumb) on the artery on the side of your windpipe (your carotid pulse) or on the radial artery near the thumb side of the wrist. Stop periodically during your workout and count your pulse rate for fifteen seconds. Multiply this number by four to get your total pulse for one minute.

Your target heart rate zone will vary depending on your age and your fitness level. To compute your heart rate zone, subtract your age from 220 and multiply this number by 60 percent. This gives you the lowest range. Now subtract your age from 220 and multiply this number by 80 percent to get your highest range.

Sample Target Heart Zone for Age 40	
LOW ZONE	220 - 40 = 180 × 60% = 108
HIGH ZONE	220 - 40 = 180 × 80% = 144

Keep an Exercise Journal

Keeping an exercise journal is important as you begin moving around more. Purchase a calendar, and record the amount and type of exercise and activity performed each day, as well as your physical response, such as difficulty breathing, shortness of breath, wheezing, or sneezing. Be sure to write down the amount and type of medication you used before, during, and after exertion. This data can help you and your doctor design a program with optimum benefit.

Build Body Efficiency

Once you are able to maintain a regular exercise program, you will be maximizing the efficiency of your body in the process of its production of energy. The next consideration is how to use that energy most efficiently.

The first approach is by *decreasing* the amount of energy required for you to perform your basic daily activities. This will allow you to have more energy left over for the other things you would like to do. Clearly, the most important factor here is to reduce the work load on the system. This includes not only your body weight but also the weight of anything that you are carrying or wearing and also the load induced by regulating your body temperature.

It is important to maintain a comfortable body temperature, not merely because it feels better but also because being too hot or too cold will stress the system. Stress occurs due to the need to produce extra energy to maintain your body temperature when you are too cold. It is also true when you are too hot as your blood vessels dilate in order to lose more heat and your heart has to beat more frequently to maintain your blood pressure. Being too hot or too cold will increase your need for oxygen. This, in turn, will increase your respiratory rate and may lead to shortness of breath.

In practical terms, if you are in a hot climate, wear a well-ventilated, wide-brimmed hat and loose-fitting, light-colored clothes. Additionally, it is important to maintain an adequate fluid intake so that you can lose heat effectively by perspiration. Drinks containing alcohol or caffeine will increase your urinary output and tend to dehydrate you and so add further stress to the situation. Similarly, avoid drinks with a high sugar or salt content as they will also use available water from your body to dilute them and so decrease the available water for perspiration and temperature control.

In cold climates, the use of the newer synthetic insulating materials in clothes that are effective and light is important to avoid adding extra weight. It is also important that these materials permit the passage of water vapor so that they do not trap perspiration between your skin and the garment. If this occurs, they first cause you to feel hot by preventing the evaporation of perspiration. After that, the perspiration wets the materials and causes them to lose their insulating qualities and you to feel cold.

Some who are sensitive to the cold and react with shortness of breath have found satisfactory protective benefits by wearing face masks made of a porous cellulose fabric. This allows more freedom to spend time out-of-doors and exercise without complaints.

In lay terms, if your clothing doesn't breathe right, then neither do you. To breathe right and feel the best you can, look after your body the best way you know how. Unlike the analogy with the motor vehicle, you can't trade yourself in next year even if you think you would be better off with the newer model.

Seek Instruction from a Therapist

Pulmonary rehabilitation would benefit those with chronic lung disease such as emphysema, chronic bronchitis, asthma, and other lung diseases. Because the symptoms are physiologic in nature, a respiratory care practitioner can help you to become more active. This professional performs procedures that are both diagnostic and therapeutic. A respiratory therapist can measure the capacity of your lungs to determine impairment, as well as perform stress tests to measure your cardiovascular strength.

After the diagnosis, the respiratory therapist will enable you to start focusing on lifestyle changes with physical conditioning activities rather than on your chronic dysfunction. Your therapist will teach you ways to reduce the symptoms and complications while improving your physical conditioning and exercise performance. You will learn how to incorporate these activities into your daily life and how to control negative reactions to stress with proper breathing and exercise.

Following your doctor's instructions, along with the suggestions in this chapter, you should be able to incorporate exercise and activity in your daily routine and help optimize your breathing capacity.

chapter 8

Using a Nutritional Approach

The idea that food and nutrition can play a key role in the prevention and treatment of many breathing problems may be hard to credit. However, fascinating evidence regarding food triggers and respiratory problems continues to surface. Some newer studies suggest that a diet high in sugar and fat may be a factor in the development of asthma among children with common allergies. Other sophisticated research has revealed that such foods as bananas, peanuts, and corn may trigger bronchoconstriction in an airway, especially when combined with exercise.

While certain foods can take your breath away, others can breathe new life into an ailing body! The latest research supports the fact that a diet rich in certain nutrients provided in food sources can help the body's immune system to function properly and lessen or even ward off infection—two important bonuses for those with chronic respiratory ailments.

Reading the Food Label

Starting with the food label is a must as you learn how nutrition affects your breathing. Especially for those who have a risk of fatal reactions to certain foods or who are sensitive to cross-reacting foods, reading labels is imperative. Although government intervention has helped to improve the information provided to the consumer, it is important to know that there are serious problems with food labels. For example, if the label says "egg substitutes," some who are allergic to eggs may think this product is safe to eat. Yet these substitutes may not have the high cholesterol egg yolks but contain egg whites, which can trigger a major allergic episode or even anaphylaxis for the egg-sensitive person. Products containing powdered sugar also contain corn starch, a by-product of corn, which can trigger reactions in those who are allergic. Nevertheless, if you read a food label, you may only find the words "powdered sugar" as ingredients present in very small amounts of foods are not required to be listed at all. For the person with potentially fatal allergies to foods such as peanuts, eggs, or corn, this misrepresentation on the label could result in a respiratory disaster.

A major problem can also occur from cross-contamination during the preparation of packaged foods. This occurs when utensils used to cook one product are reused for another product yet still have contaminants or crumbs on them. For example, enough crumbs from a peanut product may be in a mixing bowl used for a nonpeanut product to cause a dangerous reaction in the susceptible person, yet this will not be listed on a food label. If you have food allergies, always use caution when eating any new food or in a new environment.

The Food Elimination Diet

You may wonder how to tell whether a certain food causes an allergic reaction. While there are specific tests doctors can do, mounting evidence has shown that an elimination diet is most valuable in identifying allergenic foods. This diet works by eliminating the most common foods that may trigger an allergic reaction for two weeks. When symptoms subside, you slowly reintroduce these foods one at a time to see which you may be allergic to.

Some of the most common foods you eliminate at first may include:

Milk (butter, ice cream, yogurt, cheese, and other dairy products)

Wheat (breads, crackers, cookies, noodles, and other wheat products)

Corn (grits, popcorn, corn chips, corn syrups, corn starches, and other corn products)

Citrus (oranges, grapefruits, lemons, limes, and other citrus and juices)

Tomato (pizza, spaghetti sauce, catsup, and other tomato products)

Yeast (dried fruits, vinegar, mushrooms, bread, pickles, and others)

Soybean (soy sauce, soy lecithin, and tofu)

Carob (eggs, chocolate, colas, beans, peas, peanuts, and peanut butter)

Foods that are usually allowed during the elimination process include many fresh meats, vegetables, and fruits (except the listed varieties), rice cereals, and water.

After a period of strict abstinence from certain allergenic foods, you may reintroduce the foods one at a time. For example, if you are instructed to reintroduce corn, you would eat only a small amount of corn at first, as a reaction could occur. If you have no reaction with the introduced food, then you can eat this again in slightly larger amounts. You should also try by-products of the food to see if these are tolerated. If there is no change in your symptoms and the food is tolerated, with your doctor's instruction, you can go to the next category and reintroduce another food. If symptoms do develop, the new food should be stopped immediately until the symptoms clear.

Food elimination diets are to be used under the careful supervision of a physician or licensed nutritionist. You need to be sure that the remaining foods in your diet during this period supply you with adequate nutrition. Do not attempt to try these diets on your own as your body's reaction to a reintroduced allergen may be severe and require emergency medical attention.

A Word of Caution

Sulfites, which are used in foods and drugs as preservatives, can cause fatal allergic reactions in some people. Such sulfites as bisulfite, potassium, metabisulfite, sodium bisulfite, and sodium sulfite are frequently contained in many bakery products, dehydrated potatoes, corn syrup, shellfish, salad dressings, pickles, wine and beer, and dried fruits. Surprisingly, sulfites are also found in some prescription and nonprescription drugs used by those with breathing problems, including epinephrine and some nebulizers.

Some artificial colors, particularly tartrazine or yellow food dye no. 5, can be dangerous for those with allergy or asthma. Yellow food dye no. 5 may create breathing problems for those who have asthma and those who are allergic to aspirin.

If you are allergic to molds, certain foods may exacerbate your problem. Watch out for fermented foods such as beer, cider, sauerkraut, vinegar, and wine and foods made with yeast, such as breads, rolls, and many bakery products. Cheese, sour cream, buttermilk, and mushrooms can also aggravate a mold allergy.

The Benefit of Antioxidants

The role of diet in the genesis of breathing disorders is just beginning to make headlines. Evidence is accumulating that diseases, such as asthma, may have their origin in deleterious oxygen-free radical reactions. These reactions are chemical processes that change oxygen to free radicals.

In the body, free radicals can damage the proteins and fats that make up the cell membranes and DNA in cells. Considerable evidence also suggests that stress due to oxygen free radicals results in inflammation and tissue damage in the respiratory system. Immune system activation causes inflammation which damages cells by way of free radicals. Of late some studies even suggest if you have a selenium dietary deficiency, as well as low dietary intakes of vitamins C and E, you may be at higher risk for asthma or other lung problems.

Free Radicals

Somewhere along the line of reactions associated with inflammation, such as in asthma, damage associated with infection, radiation, or aging, substances called *oxygen free radicals* are formed. Cells may then leak out vital substances or dangerous chemicals that can spread destruction. Although cells usually have defense mechanisms to protect themselves from these potentially destructive chemical products, sometimes the rate of production of free radicals is great enough to overwhelm these defenses.

Free radical scavenging agents known as *antioxidants* are the main defense available to cells against the damaging effects of the free radicals. Antioxidants are enzymes that catalyze or speed up the removal of the free radicals. These enzymes contain trace nutrients such as copper, zinc, manganese, and selenium. Of the nonenzymatic agents such as vitamins E and C, the most important is vitamin E, or alpha-tocopherol, which gets into the cell membranes in human tissues to protect them from damage.

If what current research suggests is true, tissue damage in obstructive lung disease is an inflammatory phenomenon related to damage mediated by oxygen free radicals. The results of a myriad of new studies suggest that a strong free radical–antioxidant imbalance causes lung damage.

In research, free radicals have been shown to disrupt and tear apart vital cell structures like cell membranes. However, antioxidants have been shown to tie up these free radicals and take away their destructive power. This may reduce the risk of many chronic diseases, specifically lung diseases, and even slow the aging process. Eating healthful foods, including those that are high in antioxidants (beta-carotene and vitamins C and E) and phytochemicals may be helpful. Phytochemicals are substances that plants naturally produce to protect themselves against disease. They *may* help to protect us against some cancers, heart disease, and other chronic health problems. Be sure that when you prepare these supernutrients, you cook them using as little liquid as possible to prevent nutrient loss. In fact, including more raw fruits and vegetables in your diet is the best way to ensure a high intake of antioxidants and phyto-chemicals.

Understanding Antioxidant Food Sources

Vitamin A (Beta-carotene)

Vitamin A is needed to provide resistance to infections, prevent night blindness, and maintain the health of our mucosal membranes. Active vitamin A is found in animal sources like liver, fish oil, eggs, and milk fortified with vitamin A. Beta-carotene is found in apricots, carrots, cantaloupes, pumpkins, and spinach and is converted to vitamin A in the body.

Because the vitamin A found in animal sources is fat sol-uble, it can be stored in the body and, if stored in excess, can lead to toxicity symptoms such as headache, nausea, and blurred vision. On the other hand, beta-carotene, which is found in fruits and vegetables, does not seem to cause any serious side effects except skin yellowing, which goes away when you cut back on beta-carotene consumption.

If you follow the guidelines issued by most health organizations and eat five or six fruits and vegetables daily, you can easily get enough of this powerful antioxidant. For example, one quarter of a cantaloupe gives you nearly half the recommended daily requirement of beta-carotene and is a rich source of vitamin C. Spinach is not only full of beta-carotene but also contains vitamin C, folic acid, and magnesium. Be cautious when getting your beta-carotene from dried fruits as they are treated with sulfur dioxide, a chemical that can cause an asthma attack in susceptible people.

The Recommended Dietary Allowance (RDA) depends on age and sex. Current RDAs for vitamin A are 5,000 IU (International Unit) for men, and 4,000 IU for women. Although many people try to get vitamin A and beta-carotene from supplements, using natural foods is best. Because vitamin A can build up in your system, you may take too much of a supplement; this leads to toxicity. Also, your supplement may not be absorbed fully in the body, and the potency of the supplement can diminish over a period of time.

Because of a great deal of media attention, most people think of only beta-carotene as having antioxidant properties, but there are many other carotenoid compounds to choose from, including:

Carotenoid Compound	Food Sources
Alpha-caroten	Carrots, cantaloupes, and pumpkins
Beta-cryptoxanthin	Mangoes, nectarines, peaches, and tangerines
Gamma-carotene	Apricots and tomatoes
Lutein and zeaxanthin	Beets, corn, collards, and mustards
Lycopene	Guavas, pink grapefruits, tomatoes, and watermelons

Vitamin A Food Sources	
Apricots	Milk
Asparagus	Mustard greens
Beef liver	Oranges
Bell peppers, red	Papayas
Broccoli	Spinach
Cantaloupes	Sweet potatoes
Carrots	Watermelons
Eggs	Winter squash
Kale	

Vitamin C

Vitamin C (ascorbic acid) protects us against infection and aids in wound healing. When the body is under great stress, the blood levels of ascorbic acid have been found to decline. This decline also occurs with age in both men and women.

The possible influence of dietary antioxidants, especially vitamin C, on the increasing prevalence of asthma is being explored. In a comprehensive study, researchers found that vitamin C intake in the general population appears to correlate with asthma; this suggests that a diet low in vitamin C may be one risk factor for this breathing disorder. Vitamin C is the major antioxidant substance present in the airway surface liquid of the lung, where it could be important in protecting against oxidants.

Though there is still some controversy regarding vitamin C and its relationship to asthma, there is research showing that vitamin C may help to prevent shortness of breath from COPD. One study analyzed the diets and lung functions of 2,633 people and concluded that more vitamin C meant better lung function. The difference between those who ate the most vitamin C and those who took in the least was like the difference between people who smoked a pack of cigarettes a day for five to seven years and those who didn't.

While there is no direct research evaluating vitamin C in preventing colds, several studies have shown that this vitamin can markedly lessen both the symptoms and duration of a cold. These studies show that a 500-milligram tablet taken four times a day can help reduce cold symptoms.

Although the current RDA of vitamin C is only 60 milligrams, many nutritionists feel that this amount is far too low to have any benefit. While the research on increasing this amount is positive, it is still inconclusive, and each person is different. Always check with your doctor before taking additional supplements.

Vitamin C Food Sources	
Broccoli	Papayas
Cantaloupes	Red, green, or
Cauliflower	yellow peppers
Kale	Strawberries
Kiwis	Sweet potatoes
Oranges	Tomatoes

Vitamin E

Sophisticated research has found vitamin E to be a powerful antioxidant and important to the body for the maintenance of cell membranes. This vitamin's antioxidant effect may slow age-related changes of the body, and some recent studies suggest that vitamin E may be associated with lower incidences of asthma, although more research is needed to assess exactly how much vitamin E is needed.

This vitamin is taken in through vegetables and seed oils; therefore, ingesting large amounts is difficult, especially if you are following a low-fat diet. Wheat germ is a great source of vitamin E, as well as other disease-fighting nutrients such as B vitamins, magnesium, and calcium. Peanut butter and sunflower seeds are also good sources of vitamin E.

Some researchers feel that the current recommended dietary allowance for vitamin E—15 IU for men and 12 IU for women—may be too low for disease protection. Although the synthetic vitamin E found in supplements may not be as potent as the natural form found in foods, you may wish to ask your doctor whether vitamin E supplementation is necessary for you. These supplements can be purchased at grocery or health food stores and pharmacies.

Vitamin E Food Sources	
Almonds	Lobster
Corn oil	Peanut butter
Cod-liver oil	Safflower oil
Corn oil margarine	Salmon steak
Hazelnuts	Sunflower seeds

Bioflavonoids

Hosts of experiments on bioflavonoids found in the soft white skin of citrus fruits have suggested that these key nutrients may play a role in allergy treatment as they increase immune system activation. These biochemically active substances accompany vitamin C in plants and act as an antioxidant. You can find bioflavonoids in the pulp and white core that runs through the center of citrus fruits, green peppers, oranges, cherries, and grapes.

Pycnogenol

Pycnogenol, a natural antioxidant, is a special blend of water-soluble bioflavonoids and has been taken in Europe for years with no reported adverse effects. It is said to help alleviate the symptoms of hay fever and many allergies by reducing the formation of histamine and inflammation. Some studies show that pycnogenol is fifty times more potent than vitamin E and twenty times more potent than vitamin C.

Although there are no reported allergic or negative side effects of pycnogenol, again, it is most important to check with your doctor before trying pycnogenol or any supplement for that matter.

Glutathione

Another nutrient that has been found to strengthen the immune system so it can fight infections is glutathione. This powerful antioxidant is most plentiful in the red, pulpy area of the watermelon near the rind. It can also be found in brussels sprouts, spinach, broccoli, cabbage, and cauliflower.

Plant-Based Phytochemicals

Nutrition research is now revealing that a variety of food choices can do more than provide optimal nutrient intake. A varied diet can also provide hundreds of nutrient and nonnutrient compounds that may help the human body defend itself against damage, just like they help plants defend themselves against extreme weather conditions. These compounds found in plant-based foods as a group are called phytochemicals.

Phytochemicals appear in all plants, therefore a diet that includes a variety of grains, fruits, and vegetables should provide these substances. Because research confirms that a wide array of nutrients in foods, including those not yet identified, are essential for wellness, relying on supplements for good nutrition may limit your intake to just the *known* nutritional compounds rather than getting the full benefit of all nutrients in the food.

Phytochemical Food Sources	
Apples	Garlic
Apricots	Legumes
Broccoli	Onions
Brussels sprouts	Red peppers
Cabbage	Soybeans
Carrots	Sweet potatoes
Cauliflower	Tomatoes

Recommended Dietary Allowances (RDAs)

The recommended dietary allowances are issued by the Food and Nutrition Board of the National Academy of Sciences. They are the levels of nutrients thought to be adequate to meet the known nutrient needs of most healthy individuals to prevent deficiency-related diseases such as beriberi or scurvy. There is now overwhelming scientific evidence available that points to certain nutrients that should be ingested in greater amounts than the RDAs for disease prevention. For example, studies show vitamin E may protect against heart disease when taken in greater amounts than its RDA. The RDAs have not kept up with the scientific breakthroughs.

So, how do you know what foods you should eat? This is easily addressed by choosing foods from the U.S. Department of Agriculture's food guide pyramid (Figure 8.2). Choosing a variety of healthful foods from the suggested groups and focusing mainly on a variety of nutrient-dense foods and vegetables will ensure that you are getting a necessary amount of vitamins and minerals. Of course, if your eating habits are poor, you may need supplementation.

Vitamin Supplements

After reviewing the lists of key nutrients found in various foods, you may realize that your diet needs supplementation with vitamins and minerals. If you do need supplementation in your diet, start with a multiple vitamin that has the recommended dietary allowances; then talk with a registered/licensed nutritionist about your specific needs for additional vitamins and minerals. You may also ask your doctor if the following safe-dose ranges recommended by the American Medical Association's Council on Scientific Affairs would be appropriate for your situation:

Vitamin A	250 to 2,500 IU
Vitamin D	Up to 400 IU (up to age 18), Up to 200 IU (adults)
Vitamin E	6 to 30 IU
Thiamin	1 to 2 mg
Riboflavin	1 to 2 mg
Vitamin B6	1.5 to 2.5 mg
Folic acid	100 to 250 mcg
Vitamin B12	3 to 10 mg
Vitamin C	50 to 100 mg

Other Important Nurtrients to Consider

Magnesium

Magnesium appears to play a key role in a number of biochemical reactions that are important to lung function.

Although recommended dosages of magnesium range from 280 milligrams for women and 350 milligrams for men, some recent studies have found that a low intake of magnesium in the diet increases bronchial reactivity and results in asthma and chronic obstructive airways disease. These studies show that magnesium supplementation reduces bronchial constriction as well as the pressure in pulmonary arteries in cases of pulmonary hypertension. It may increase the force of the respiratory muscles. As such, magnesium may have a powerful influence over lung function with several antiasthmatic actions, as it may relax airway smooth muscle with a resultant dilation of bronchioles and also reduce airway inflammation. Although magnesium has been used in the past to treat acute asthma, there is scientific opinion that in the future, magnesium could help to prevent this disease, as well.

Magnesium Food Sources	
Almonds	Peanut butter
Artichokes	Pecans
Avocado	Pineapples
Bananas	Plantains
Black-eyed peas, dried or cooked	Raisins
Cashews	Shredded wheat
Dairy products	Soy flour
Kidney beans, dried or cooked	Soybeans, dried
Lima beans, dried or raw	Spinach
Oatmeal	Tofu
	Walnuts
	Whole wheat flour

Selenium

This mineral also operates as an antioxidant and has the function of protecting red blood cells from accumulating hydrogen peroxide—a type of free radical produced by leukocytes, white blood cells that may destroy other cells in your body. Vitamin E appears to work positively with selenium in this capacity.

The RDA is 55 micrograms for women and 70 micrograms for men. Foods high in selenium include seafood, liver, and kidney, as well as other meats.

Zinc

Zinc also has antioxidant effects and is vital to the body's resistance to infection and for tissue repair. Many illnesses, such as some cancers, kidney disease, long-term infection, trauma, and cirrhosis of the liver, are associated with zinc deficiency. Medications may also interfere with absorption in the intestines and cause a zinc deficiency.

There are exciting studies of late that suggest sucking on zinc-gluconate lozenges at the start of a cold may lessen its severity. One study at Dartmouth College reported that students who took zinc lozenges at the onset of a cold had only five days of symptoms compared with nine days for students who received placebos. This may be because zinc has an antiviral effect in the mouth and nose. Researchers from Wayne State University School of Medicine have suggested that zinc fosters immunity. The body may be unable to fight infection without sufficient supplies of this nutrient.

Other research suggests that zinc can help to improve the immune system in elderly people. However, cautions must be raised as high doses of zinc are toxic and may, in fact, suppress the immune function. Again, check with your physician for what is safe in your situation.

The RDA for zinc for women is 12 milligrams and for men 15 milligrams. Foods high in zinc include seafood, eggs, meats, whole grains, wheat germ, nuts, and seeds; tea and coffee may hinder absorption.

Controlling Your Weight

Obesity is a common impediment for those with respiratory disorders. Although about one-half of those with COPD eventually experience weight loss without an obvious cause, obesity is still a threat to millions. Even with asthma, additional weight can aggravate respiratory symptoms because the extra body fat must have oxygen. With a greatly stressed respiratory system, this added weight makes breathing more difficult. Particularly when the weight and mass of the abdomen and chest increase, breathing becomes more difficult as the diaphragm has to push down against a heavy abdomen.

Food is fuel. When you eat a nutritional, well-balanced diet, many other factors fall in place. For example, good nutrition helps maintain the ventilatory functions of the lungs. Likewise, poor nutrition can cause wasting of the diaphragm and other pulmonary muscles. Foods that are nutrient dense help fight infections and may help to prevent illness.

Just how much should you weigh? Your weight can depend on many variables, including height, age, bone structure, and weight-cycling history. The best weight for you is the one at which you have the fewest symptoms and is the closest to the recommended "normal" level. The target weight ranges for men and women given in Figure 8.1 are statistical indicators. This chart represents a way of comparing your weight to that of people who live longest at your height and body type. Work with your doctor or registered/licensed dietitian and find the weight that is best for you.

fig. 8.1 Metropolitan Height and Weight Tables

MEN[a]

| HEIGHT | | SMALL | MEDIUM | LARGE |
FEET	INCHES	FRAME	FRAME	FRAME
5	2	128–134	131–141	138–150
5	3	130–136	133–143	140–153
5	4	132–138	135–145	142–156
5	5	134–140	137–148	144–160
5	6	136–142	139–151	146–164
5	7	138–145	142–154	149–168
5	8	140–148	145–157	152–172
5	9	142–151	148–160	155–176
5	10	144–154	151–163	158–180
5	11	146–157	154–166	161–184
6	0	149–160	157–170	164–188
6	1	152–164	160–174	168–192
6	2	155–168	164–178	172–197
6	3	158–172	167–182	176–202
6	4	162–176	171–187	181–207

[a] Weights at ages 25–59 based on lowest mortality. Weight in pounds according to frame (in indoor clothing weighing 5 pounds). Height in shoes with 1-inch heels.

Metropolitan Height and Weight Tables

WOMEN[b]

| HEIGHT | | SMALL | MEDIUM | LARGE |
FEET	INCHES	FRAME	FRAME	FRAME
4	10	102–111	109–121	118–131
4	11	103–113	111–123	120–134
5	0	104–115	113–126	122–137
5	1	106–118	115–129	125–140
5	2	108–121	118–132	128–143
5	3	111–124	121–135	131–147
5	4	114–127	124–138	134–151
5	5	117–130	127–141	137–155
5	6	120–133	130–144	140–159

Metropolitan Height and Weight Tables (cont.)				
WOMEN[b]				
HEIGHT		SMALL	MEDIUM	LARGE
FEET	INCHES	FRAME	FRAME	FRAME
5	7	123–136	133–147	143–163
5	8	126–139	136–150	146–167
5	9	129–142	139–153	149–170
5	10	132–145	142–156	152–173
5	11	135–148	145–159	155–176
6	0	138–151	148–162	158–179

[b] Weights at ages 25–59 based on lowest mortality. Weight in pounds according to frame (in indoor clothing weighing 3 pounds). Height in shoes with 1-inch heels.

Calories Do Count

Not surprisingly, calories still count although selecting low-fat and nutrient-dense choices is the key to weight reduction. If you find you must reduce your weight, the American Dietetic Association recommends a calorie level of *no less than ten times your* **desired** *weight*. Women should get at least 1,200 calories, and men at least 1,400 calories a day. This is good news if you have tried to maintain a very low calorie diet with little success. For example, if your goal is 140 pounds, you should eat around 1,400 calories a day. If your goal is 180 pounds, then you can follow a diet of 1,800 calories a day for weight reduction. This daily calorie allowance will not allow a quick reduction of weight, but studies show that it is better to make lifestyle changes and lose weight slowly to make the adjustment less stressful. Gradual behavior modification is more likely to be successful especially in terms of keeping your weight under control after the initial weight loss.

Burning It Off		
CALORIES PER HOUR BURNED BY VARIOUS ACTIVITIES		
ACTIVITY	MALE (180 LB)	FEMALE (130 LB)
Carpentry	270	195
Cycling (10 mph)	486	351
Dancing (disco)	468	338
Golf (walking)	411	299
Hiking (hilly)	648	468
Jogging (6 mph)	756	546
Jumping rope	684	494
Mopping	306	221
Raking	270	195
Rowing machine	558	403
Skiing (cross country)	666	481
Snow shoveling (light)	702	502
Swimming (slow crawl)	630	455
Tennis (singles)	522	377
Trimming hedges	378	273
Walking (2–2.5 mph)	288	208
Weeding	360	260
Weight training	342	247
Window cleaning	288	208

You should understand that weight loss is more likely to occur if the calorie intake is close to or less than the caloric demands of baseline body function and activity. Keep in mind that a large amount of exercise is needed to burn up calories. For example, a man weighing 180 pounds who jogs at 6 miles per hour for one hour will burn off 756 calories. If he eats a double burger and fries at a local fast food restaurant for lunch after his run, he has taken in approximately 800 calories, or more than he burned off initially. This is not the way to lose weight! Calorie counting is essential in controlling the intake of excessive calories and managing a normal weight.

What about Weight Loss?

As stated, abnormal weight loss is a common nutritional problem with some people. If you have COPD, you may experience a progressive reduction in weight possibly due to recurrent infections which reduce the appetite and hinder eating. Also you may expend extra energy in the act of breathing. The ventilatory muscles that must work against increased resistance to airflow in the bronchial tubes can require up to ten times the calories required for a well person's muscles. Some medications you might take for infection or for breathing disorders can upset your stomach, cause nausea, and reduce appetite. Finally, the depression that is often associated with respiratory problems can reduce appetite to the point of unhealthy weight loss.

When you lose weight, the body compensates for the lack of nutrients and energy by breaking down its own

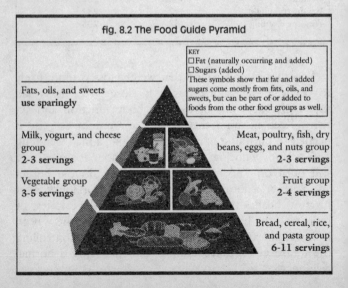

fig. 8.2 The Food Guide Pyramid

KEY
☐ Fat (naturally occurring and added)
☐ Sugars (added)
These symbols show that fat and added sugars come mostly from fats, oils, and sweets, but can be part of or added to foods from the other food groups as well.

Fats, oils, and sweets
use sparingly

Milk, yogurt, and cheese group
2-3 servings

Meat, poultry, fish, dry beans, eggs, and nuts group
2-3 servings

Vegetable group
3-5 servings

Fruit group
2-4 servings

Bread, cereal, rice, and pasta group
6-11 servings

muscle and internal organs to meet its needs. Therefore, muscle loss and muscle wasting must be prevented.

If you have a poor appetite during times of respiratory problems and cannot eat much food at one time, make sure that the food you do eat is very nutritious and high in protein. Your dietary goal should be to start out eating an adequate balanced diet including the suggested foods on the food guide pyramid (Figure 8.2) and then add to this diet from the suggestions given below.

1. Have at least two servings of milk or milk products daily such as ice cream, pudding, flavored yogurt, or cheese if you have no problems such as lactose deficiency or increased mucus production associated with dairy products.

2. Eat at least two to three servings of fruit or fruit juice every day. Include one serving of a fruit with vitamin C like oranges, guavas, strawberries, or grapefruit.

3. Include at least two to three servings of vegetables a day, including a good vitamin A source found in yellow or green leafy vegetables such as spinach.

4. Eat at least two servings of lean meat, poultry, lentils, or fish daily.

5. Include four or more servings of bread and cereal.

6. Include nutritious snacks like cheese, peanut butter, nuts, and yogurt as desired to boost protein intake.

7. Eat six mini-meals a day instead of three large ones. This will help avoid filling your stomach too much, causing shortness of breath because of the impairment of diaphragm movement.

8. Consider a nasal cannula (a small plastic tube connected to the oxygen source which delivers oxygen

through the nostrils) during mealtime if you are using oxygen.

Watch Salt Intake

Interestingly, salt intake may be related to some breathing disorders. Preliminary research suggests that dietary salt restriction in asthmatic patients results in a possible improvement of symptoms and a less frequent usage of bronchodilators. If you have lung disease, too much sodium can cause you to retain fluids that may interfere with your heart function and cause congestion in your lungs.

How much salt is enough? According to a U.S. Department of Agriculture survey, the average American consumes an average of 6,400 milligrams of sodium each day. That is the amount of salt in 1 tablespoon, but it is two and a half times the recommended daily maximum of 2,400 milligrams. The body's needs are only about ½ to 1½ teaspoons of salt a day (1,100 to 3,300 milligrams of sodium). Although the words *salt* and *sodium* are often used interchangeably, they are not the same. Ordinary table salt is only 40 percent sodium. Too much sodium can increase fluid retention and elevate blood pressure in people who are sodium sensitive.

Many foods naturally contain sodium, including animal products like meat, fish, poultry, milk, and eggs. Vegetable products are naturally low in sodium. Most of the sodium in our diets, however, comes from commercially processed foods such as cured meats like bacon and ham, luncheon meats, sausage, frozen breaded meats, fish and seafood, and canned meats and vegetables. Condiments like catsup, mustard, and steak sauce are also high in sodium. Fast foods such as hamburgers and French fries and prepare-at-home fast foods like frozen pizza, hot dogs, sausage, creamed chipped beef, and broccoli with cheese sauce are very high in sodium.

It is a good idea to reduce the salt in your diet to prevent high blood pressure, fluid retention, and possible worsening of respiratory problems. Reading the ingredient list on the label of a package to determine the sodium content is very helpful to stay within recommended limits.

Medication, Nutrition, and Digestion

Medication plays a vital role in the prevention, treatment, and management of breathing problems. Many people are living longer and more productive lives due to medication. However, serious problems may result when medicine is not taken as directed. Reactions to a medication can often seem worse than the breathing disorder it is intended to treat. For example, you may find that theophylline or oral steroids cause stomach irritation. Theophylline may cause the reflux of stomach acid in the esophagus as it relaxes the valve between the stomach and esophagus.

How Medications Interfere

Cause a poor or uncontrollable appetite.
Enhance or hinder the body's absorption of vitamins and minerals and other nutrients.
Change the way the body uses vitamins and minerals and other nutrients.
Change the rate at which the body gets rid of vitamins and minerals and other nutrients.

Be Aware of Interactions

By being aware of possible food-drug interactions that occur with your medications, you can minimize the adverse effects. Food can influence the absorption of your medication; whether your stomach is full or empty can decrease, delay, or even increase the absorption of your medication. So it is wise to know how a medication should be taken. Certain drugs such as the antibiotic azithromycin should be taken on an empty stomach to enhance their absorption into the bloodstream. Other drugs such as the antibiotics doxycycline and clarithromycin, or steroids like prednisone should be taken with food in the stomach to prevent irritation or stomach upset.

Before accepting any medication from your pharmacist, inform her or him of any other medication you are on, past reactions to medications, and your medical history—current or previous conditions—such as heart disease, high blood pressure, diabetes, or kidney disease. Carefully read and adhere to any instructions or warnings that appear on the label.

Increased Wellness

Including nutritious foods in your daily diet is one important way you can take control and help to improve your respiratory problem and add to your increased wellness and quality of life. Take notes of your past and current food intake, and then see how you can creatively include more foods packed with vitamins, minerals, antioxidants, and phytochemicals. Consider asking your doctor for a referral to a certified nutritionist for more specific dietary information to help you stay well.

chapter 9

Controlling Nighttime Problems

On a normal day, we rarely *think* about breathing. Breathing is one of those bodily functions that happens by itself. We trust that our internal control systems function normally so our breathing continues day or night, awake or asleep, no matter what.

But how this changes when we are ill! Respiration then becomes the full focus of our attention, and we become acutely aware of each breath. Problems with the respiratory system can be so upsetting that we find it difficult to fall asleep or to stay asleep. Our periods of sleep, which we have come to appreciate as times to rest, relax, and rejuvenate, can instead become torturous, anxious, and exhausting.

The Sleep Robbers

What disturbs your sleep? A badly congested nose or mucus dripping down a sore throat can be intruding. Chest tightness, shortness of breath, or other difficulty breathing can make sleep impossible. A hacking cough causes frequent wakenings. Various sleep-related breathing disorders can fragment and ruin sleep and leave us unrefreshed and sleepy throughout the following day.

John, a forty-nine-year-old computer sales associate, had suffered with interrupted sleep for years due to his thunderous snoring problem. His nighttime snoring worsened to the point that his wife moved her sleeping quarters to the other side of their home to get a full night's rest. However, what particularly frightened her were the episodes of breath holding (apneic spells) John experienced during his sleep. These lasted up to one minute each. She was also concerned about his inability to stay awake at family functions, during sermons, or in the movie theater. John was personally concerned about his severe headaches that occurred every morning, when he dragged his fatigued body to the kitchen for his first large mug of coffee.

When his teenage daughter read about sleep apnea in a popular magazine, she encouraged her parents to go to a sleep disorders center for help. After a series of consultations and sleep testing, John found out that he did have sleep apnea. Symptoms of sleep apnea are discussed in detail on pages 199–202 and include loud, annoying snoring that is punctuated by quiet spells (cessation of breathing, called apneas). These apneas are ended by an audible resumption of breathing and continuation of snoring.

John soon discovered that a close business colleague had the same problem and was successfully treated with a nasal continuous positive airway pressure (CPAP) (page 205). This is a custom-fit mask placed over the nose with a tight-fitting seal. It is attached by a flexible hose to a pump that quietly produces a positive pressure within the upper airway to keep the airway from collapsing.

John used the nasal CPAP for a short time and was amazed at how much better he felt. His headaches soon disappeared, and his alertness and energy level increased.

His wife even moved back into their bedroom because he no longer snored. Also, his hunting buddies agreed that John could rejoin the group, but only if he brought along his portable battery system to run his CPAP machine at the campsite.

John is now a committed "sleep activist" and speaks regularly at support groups for people with sleep apnea, telling them of new treatments that can change their lives.

Millions like John have sought help for respiratory problems which hindered restful sleep. To understand how breathing problems affect sleep, you must know what normal sleep is.

Normal Sleep: Time and Stages

Normal adults generally sleep seven to eight hours each night. Some may require more, and some get by quite well with much less. Newborn babies generally need sixteen or seventeen hours of sleep each day with about eight hours during the night and about eight during daylight hours divided into many naps. With maturation, the child spends an increased amount of time asleep at night and less time napping during the day. By age four, the preschool child is sleeping about ten to twelve hours a night without any naps. Then, with age, there is a gradual decrease in nighttime sleep down to the adult quota.

Current evidence now suggests that a complex of nerve cells and interconnections called a *circadian pacemaker* within the brain are responsible for the cycles of sleep and wakefulness. Under normal circumstances, you will awaken in the morning in response to some cue such as an alarm clock or sunlight beaming through your bedroom window. As the morning hours advance, you get more alert until about 1 or 2 P.M. when you have a lull or sag in wakefulness. Although many think this dip in alertness is due to a heavy lunch, this is not so. The lull is a natural consequence of your circadian rhythm. Later in the afternoon your alertness improves again until late evening when you start to experience a wave of sleepiness. With your usual bedtime ritual, you will fall asleep until the next morning when the cycle starts again.

Problems in your cycle arise when snoring or a respiratory infection ruin sleep and cause a more pronounced afternoon droop. Usually, these disorders diminish your alertness through the entire cycle.

Distinct Stages of Sleep

Sleep is made up of distinct stages with specific characteristics defined by brain waves, eye movements, and muscle tension. In a sleep lab, these stages are recorded by electroencephalography (EEG), electrooculogram (EOG), and electromyogram (EMG), as defined on page 189. The two broad categories of sleep include rapid eye movement (REM) and nonrapid eye movement (NREM) sleep.

During REM sleep, there are small, variable-speed brain waves, rapid eye movements like those of eyes-open wakefulness, and absent muscle tension in all muscles except those needed to breathe such as the diaphragm. It is during REM sleep that you have most of your dreams. Arousals from this stage of sleep are usually associated with recalls of vivid imagery.

After the first few months of life, NREM sleep differentiates into four stages. These are stages I, II, II, and IV and are characterized by different combinations of brain waves, eye movements, and reduced muscle tension. The stages of NREM sleep vary from drowsiness to very deep sleep. If you have ever been confused or disoriented when someone awoke you, you were probably in stage III or IV sleep.

Throughout the night, you cycle through NREM sleep stages I to IV and REM sleep about every ninety minutes.

In the early part of the night's sleep period, there is more NREM stage III and IV sleep. Closer to morning awakening, there is more REM sleep. Various respiratory problems may disrupt this normal pattern of sleep and cause you to feel unrefreshed in the morning.

Electroencephalography uses an apparatus for recording electrical activity from the brain. It uses special electrodes or probes placed on the scalp attached by wires to an amplifier which can convert the electrical signals to wavelike written forms on papers or to images on a computer screen.

Electrooculogram records the electrical voltage that exists between the front and back of the eye. This particular electrical activity changes along with eye movement and is detected by electrodes placed on the skin near the eye. Movements of the eye appear as tracings on paper or screen.

Electromyogram involves an instrument that converts electrical activity associated with functioning muscle into a written or visual record. Higher muscle tension appears as a thicker line on this recording.

Sleep and Breathing Patterns

Sleep modifies the depth of your breaths and your rate of breathing. It also affects your respiratory responses to changes in oxygen or carbon dioxide levels in the blood or to changes in airway resistance. Unlike your heart, the respiratory muscles do not have a built-in pacemaker. Rather, they depend on nerve signals from the respiratory center in the part of the brainstem known as the *medulla*. The medulla receives and processes input related to changes in oxygen, carbon dioxide, and acid content in the blood. It also processes mechanical information from the lung or chest wall and behavioral information from the higher brain centers.

When you first fall asleep, there is a normal pattern of waxing and waning of breathing amplitude called *peri-*

odic breathing. There are also some apneas (cessation-of-breathing events) during drowsiness called *central type*.

In NREM sleep, your breathing will be remarkably regular. Yet, there is a tendency for the speed of breathing inspiration (breathing in) to be decreased as you go into progressively deeper stages of NREM sleep. There is also an increase in upper airway resistance at the base of the tongue toward the back of the throat. This resistance occurs because of fewer nerve signals sent to muscles in that region of the body. When you are awake and active, these nerve signals keep the airway open. This lack of synchrony between the upper airway muscles and the muscles of the respiratory pump can predispose you to obstructive sleep apnea that involves narrowing of the airway and blockage of the airflow.

During NREM sleep, you will have a *decrease* in the tendency to breathe harder and deeper compared to your breathing response during wakefulness. This reduction in breathing response can prolong the length of time that decreased airflow through the upper airway occurs.

Breathing during REM sleep is irregular. You will experience sudden variability in both the size and frequency of breaths. You may also have central apneas (cessations of breathing) that last ten to thirty seconds. These sudden changes occur just when there are bursts of rapid eye movements. The rib cage contribution to breathing during REM sleep is decreased because of reduced activity of the muscles between the ribs. For those with emphysema or bronchitis, this may result in smaller lung volumes and resultant low oxygen levels.

Also, during REM sleep, diaphragm activity is increased. The muscles that keep the upper airway open are almost completely relaxed. Obstructive sleep apnea may be most severe during REM sleep.

The main goal of the respiratory system is to keep the blood levels of oxygen, carbon dioxide, and acid in a compatible range with normal functions of the body and its cells. Therefore, as oxygen levels fall or carbon dioxide levels rise, the rate of breathing will increase at an appropriate pace on demand. However, during sleep, the reaction to low levels of oxygen or high levels of carbon dioxide is not as responsive. This unresponsiveness is even more pronounced when a respiratory disease causes breathing abnormalities.

During times of increased airway resistance, such as asthma or sleep apnea, you will have a tendency to awaken. Arousal from REM sleep is easier than from deep NREM sleep. Because sleep inhibits the normal gag reflexes, you have a greater risk of aspirating mucus from the nose or sinuses or even regurgitated stomach contents during deep sleep, which can result in aspiration pneumonia. Sleep also *reduces* cough, which occurs as a reaction to inhaled irritants even in normal people.

Circadian Rhythms and Diseases

During the twenty-four-hour day, the human body varies in its cycles of wakefulness and sleep. The cyclic changes you experience cause day/night differences in your susceptibility or resistance to diseases and to the severity of symptoms. For example, allergic rhinitis with sneezing, runny nose, or nasal congestion is typically worse on awakening in the morning than during the middle of an active day. If you have allergies, you are less likely to have positive tests for allergy if these tests are done in the morning compared with later in the day. In fact, the tendency to react to skin tests (see page 78) with the usual redness or hardening of the skin will be less during the morning hours than it would be in the evening or before bedtime when it is the greatest.

Sleep-Related Asthma and Treatment

Asthma receives much attention because it is a potentially disabling disease and powerfully influenced by circadian rhythms. The chances of asthma symptoms are one hundred times higher during sleep. Your asthma symptoms of nocturnal wheezing, cough, and trouble breathing are common yet potentially dangerous. Many doctors often underestimate nocturnal asthma because most medical clinics are open during the day and testing is done on awake patients.

Scientists have realized that people with asthma have a set circadian rhythm. Simple measures of expiratory airflow from the lungs through the bronchial tubes (spirometry or peak flow) are significantly higher around midday or in the afternoon than overnight or in the morning on arising. If you monitor your peak flow rate, your afternoon maximum airflow, when compared with your morning minimum, may show a 25 percent variation if you have mild asthma. In severe cases, the variation may be as high as 60 percent. Generally, the more unstable and severe the asthma, the greater the variation in flow rates.

A survey of almost 8,000 patients with asthma who were treated in primary care clinics in the United Kingdom showed that about 40 percent complained of awakening every night and almost all had nocturnal symptoms at least once a month. Among the 3,000 patients who considered their asthma mild, 25 percent were awakened with symptoms each night in spite of the medicines they were taking. In another study of about 3,000 asthmatics, approximately 90 percent reported symptoms between 10 P.M. and 7 A.M., while the reported peak incidence of symptoms was at 4 A.M.

With asthma, your bronchial flows, symptoms, and pulmonary function test results are affected by the *time of day*. If your asthma is stable, your response to bronchodilators will usually follow a circadian rhythm. This means that the effects of these drugs are *stronger when inhaled in the morning or evening* but not as strong around noontime. This variation could greatly affect any test results. In fact, morning tests are more likely to represent true reversibility of the airway obstruction. Those done around midday are likely to underestimate the amount of reversibility in bronchial obstruction.

Studies done over the last twenty years show that most deaths related to asthma occur at night. Nocturnal asthma attacks can cause significant problems sleeping, resulting in sleep deprivation and daytime sleepiness, fatigue, and irritability. These problems may affect your quality of life overall and may make it more difficult to control daytime asthma.

The exact reasons why asthma is worse during sleep are not known, but many explanations are possible. Some of these involve increased exposure to allergens at night, cooling of the airways, reclining position, or hormone secretions that follow a circadian pattern. Sleep itself may even cause changes in bronchial function.

If you are exposed to an allergen, the chances are great that airway obstruction will occur shortly afterward. This acute reaction ends within one hour. About 50 percent of those who experience an immediate reaction also have a second phase of airway obstruction within three to eight hours of exposure to the allergen. This phase, which was discussed on page 16, is known as the *late-phase response*. It is characterized by an increase in airway responsiveness, development of bronchial inflammation, and a more prolonged period of airway obstruction.

Many studies report that when allergen exposure occurs in the evening instead of in the morning, you are more susceptible to having a late-phase response and are more likely to have one of greater severity. Occasionally, one episode of exposure can cause recurring nighttime asthma symptoms for several days after.

Asthma problems may occur during sleep regardless of when the sleep period is taking place. People with asthma who work on the night shift may have breathing attacks during the day when they are sleeping. Correlations between exact sleep stages and the worsening of asthma have not been found, but most research suggests that spirometry measurements are worse about four to six hours after you fall asleep. This suggests there may be some internal trigger for sleep-related asthma.

Lying in a reclining position may also predispose you to nighttime asthma problems. Many factors may cause this such as the accumulation of secretions in the airways, increased blood volume in the lungs, decreased lung volumes, and increased airway resistance.

Breathing colder air at night or in an air-conditioned bedroom may also cause loss of heat from the airways. Airway cooling and moisture loss are considered important triggers of exercise-induced asthma. They are also implicated in nighttime asthma.

If you are frequently bothered with heartburn, the reflux of stomach acid up through the esophagus to the larynx may stimulate a reflex associated with a bronchial spasm. This reflux is worse when you lie down and if you take medicines for asthma that relax the valve between the stomach and the esophagus. Sometimes, acid from the stomach will irritate the lower esophagus and may activate the vagus nerve, which sends signals to the bronchial tubes that result in bronchoconstriction. If acidic gastric juice regurgitates all the way up the esophagus to the back of the throat and some of it drips down into the trachea, bronchi, and lungs, a severe reaction may take place. This can involve airway irritation, increased mucus production, and bronchoconstriction. In some cases, a severe type of chemical pneumonia may result.

Hormones that circulate in the blood have well-characterized circadian rhythms which are seen in those with asthma and also those without asthma. Epinephrine is one such hormone, which exerts important influences on the bronchial tubes. This hormone helps keep the muscle in the walls of the bronchi relaxed so the airway remains wide. It also suppresses the release of other substances, such as histamine, which cause mucus secretion and bronchospasm. Your epinephrine levels and peak expiratory flow rates are lowest at about 4 A.M., while histamine levels tend to peak at this time. This decrease in epinephrine level may predispose you to an asthma attack.

Since sleep-related asthma may occur anytime during the sleep period, treatment must be sufficient to cover these hours. Long-acting bronchodilators are available as pills (theophylline) or inhaled medication (salmeterol). Both are effective in preventing bronchospasm. If you suffer from sleep-related asthma, you will also find great benefit from a long-acting inhaled corticosteroid taken close to sleep time. For those who have gastroesophageal reflux problems, a medicine that reduces acid secretions from the stomach will also be helpful at sleep time. Avoidance of potential allergy triggering items such as feathers in down pillows or comforters may also be very helpful in preventing sleep-related asthma attacks.

Snoring and Treatment

We cannot discuss nighttime breathing problems without addressing a main concern—snoring. Snoring is a common nuisance that is due to changes in the upper airway from the back of the nose to the base of the tongue at the level of the larynx (voice box), which occur during sleep.

The snoring sound itself is produced by the vibration of

the soft tissues of the soft palate, pharynx, and uvula. Snoring occurs as you breathe in and out and may be heard whether you breathe exclusively through your nose or mouth or through both your nose and mouth at the same time.

Snoring is very common, especially as we age. One study found that men have a higher incidence of snoring (25 percent) compared with women (15 percent); older people snore more than younger people. Snoring increases in both sexes after the age of thirty-five, and while it remains stable in women, it slowly diminishes in men after age sixty-five. An astounding 60 percent of men and 40 percent of women between ages forty-one and sixty-five are habitual snorers. It has been said that our primitive ancestors snored loudly to frighten away predators. Now snoring is recognized as a threat to the success of many marriages and to our health.

Obnoxious snoring has disturbed the sleep of bed partners and others nearby for millennia. In fact, the bed partner or family members can provide important information regarding the loudness, frequency, and factors that worsen the snoring such as position (lying on back or side). Remedies have varied from sleeping with the mouth closed by a cloth or other device to more dramatic ones. The gunslinger John Wesley Hardin is said to have fatally shot a loud snorer sleeping in the next room!

Common Risk Factors for Snoring
Male gender
Obesity
Alcohol ingestion
Use of tranquilizers, muscle relaxants, or sleeping pills
Smoking cigarettes

The prominence of snoring in men may be due to differences between men and women in hormonal influences on the upper airway muscles, deposition of fat, and the anatomy of the upper airway. A mere glass or two of wine with supper, especially if consumed late or close to bedtime, will aggravate snoring. Drugs that tend to sedate the nervous system like alcohol cause increased relaxation of the pharyngeal muscles during sleep with more of a tendency to vibrate as air passes in and out. Smoking may worsen snoring by causing irritation, inflammation, and swelling of the throat with resultant narrowing.

Nasal obstruction whether due to a deviated septum, polyps, or seasonal or perennial allergies may exacerbate snoring by increasing the resistance to airflow through the upper airway. Some individuals with a small or backward-positioned jawbone may be predisposed to snoring because of the crowding of the airspace at the base of the tongue.

Since snoring is so common, it was once considered normal and a mere social problem. However, in the early 1970s studies suggested that snoring might be more than a noisy distraction. It became clear that high blood pressure, coronary artery disease, and strokes are more frequent among habitual snorers. Further research has pointed out that it is not snoring itself that causes the health consequences but other puzzling factors.

Sometimes snoring is a symptom of a much more serious condition known as *obstructive sleep apnea* which involves very severe narrowing of the upper airway during sleep. The narrowing may be complete with occlusion of the airway and cessation of airflow. Patients with obstructive sleep apnea not only snore but have other symptoms after what they thought was a good night's sleep.

Depending on the group of people studied, 10 to 50 percent of individuals who snore have obstructive sleep apena. Also, up to 67 percent of people who have obstructive sleep apnea are overweight. Analysis of data from several studies suggests that the association between snoring and high blood pressure, coronary disease, and strokes may be due to obesity and the presence of obstructive sleep apnea.

Identifying the type of snoring you have is important. You may have *primary* or "pure" snoring if you snore but do *not* have:

Significant reductions in air flow through the back of the throat to the lungs

Decreases in oxygen levels in the blood

Excessive daytime sleepiness or other symptoms due to sleep disruption

If you have pure snoring, you can take some steps today to reduce this. If you are overweight, losing down to your recommended weight can help you reduce snoring. Drug therapy and dental appliances for pulling the tongue or jawbone forward may be helpful. These therapies will be discussed in more detail on pages 202 to 205.

Sometimes, surgery to open blocked passages in the nose may be helpful. A number of different devices designed to open the nose such as internal dilators or external strips for dilating the nostrils are available in many grocery and drugstores. While studies have shown individual improvement in breathing or sleepiness, there is no consistent objective data to show an improvement in snoring or sleep quality when these are used.

Surgery or more recently laser-assisted surgery on the upper airway is helpful to reduce the size of the uvula and soft palate. This helps to reduce the source of the snoring sounds. The laser surgery can be done with local anesthesia in an ear, nose, and throat doctor's office. Of course, be sure that you check the credentials, training, and experience of the surgeon with your own doctor and also with the county medical society. Also make sure that your snoring is not associated with obstructive sleep apnea because surgery is not a dependable way to treat this problem.

If you suffer from snoring and sleep apnea, there is no accurate or reliable way to predict whether you will respond successfully to the surgery. You may run the risk of going from being someone with sleep apnea who snores to being someone who still has sleep apnea but no longer has the key noisy signal (snoring).

It is important that you have proper sleep studies for snoring if you are considering surgery. To make sure that snoring is not a symptom of obstructive sleep apnea, special sleep studies, called *polysomnography* (see page 202), are done. Your doctor can see whether these are required for your situation.

Signs and Symptoms of Obstructive Sleep Apnea

In adults, obstructive sleep apnea is more common than asthma. The most common complaint or symptom related to obstructive sleep apnea is loud, annoying snoring that is punctuated by quiet spells (cessations of breathing called apneas). These apneas end with an audible resumption of breathing and continuation of snoring. A brief arousal also occurs at the end of apneas and can be measured by brain wave recordings.

The intrusions of wakefulness during sleep or shifts in sleep stages (from a deep stage to one that is less deep) frequently result in fragmented sleep and sleep deprivation. If you experience these, you may also complain of excessive daytime sleepiness. Some people are even unaware of daytime sleepiness because they do not perceive their own problem due to the lack of quality sleep.

Daytime sleepiness has been estimated to occur in 5 percent of the population, and of these people, 30 to 40 percent have obstructive sleep apnea. Sleepiness is particularly likely to be evident in situations which are monotonous or in which there is little stimulation such as sitting alone, reading, watching television, taking long car rides, or listening to lectures or sermons. A simple questionnaire known as the *Epworth Sleepiness Scale* (see page 203) is used by some sleep medicine experts for evaluating the tendency to doze off during the day. This questionnaire was developed by Dr. Murray Johns and involves assigning a number to the likelihood of falling asleep in certain circumstances. A total score above seven is considered abnormal. The higher the score, the more likely you will doze off.

It is important to note that behavior may compensate for physiologic sleepiness. A highly motivated person working at a demanding job may not complain of being sleepy. Some folks drink large amounts of caffeinated beverages and may be compensating for their tendency to doze off during the day. Indeed, the Epworth Sleepiness Scale score must be interpreted in light of how much stimulant the person takes in a day.

Those with sleep apnea who have excessive daytime sleepiness as a prominent symptom may be mistakenly labeled as *narcoleptics*. Narcoleptics classically have cataplexy (loss of muscle tone when angry, surprised, or amused), sleep paralysis (loss of muscle tone on drifting off to sleep or on awakening), and hypnagogic hallucinations (vivid dreams that occur at going to sleep). Special sleep studies can distinguish obstructive sleep apnea from narcolepsy.

With obstructive sleep apnea, you may suffer from symptoms such as restless sleep (extra movements at the end of apnea spells), morning headaches, sore throat, dry mouth, cough, personality change (depression, moodiness, irritability), sexual impotence, and frequent awakenings throughout the night. You may also awaken several times during the night to urinate and attribute this to urological problems, when the cause of your sleep disruption is sleep apnea. Without the sleep-related breathing disorder, chances are great that you would sleep through the night and empty your bladder in the morning on arising.

Interestingly, high blood pressure is common in those with obstructive sleep apnea. In fact, obstructive sleep apnea has been observed in 20 to 30 percent of people with hypertension. Increases in systolic and diastolic blood pressures that correlate with decreases in oxygen levels in the blood are associated with apneas. Blood pressure normally falls during NREM deep sleep because of the dilation of the blood vessels. However, this normal dilation with blood pressure decrease does not occur in people with sleep apnea. For many, there may be vasoconstriction and elevation in blood pressure which can carry over to waking hours.

Nasal obstruction due to polyps or a deviated septum, or swelling or enlargement of the tonsils or adenoids may increase the risk of obstructive sleep apnea. A long palate or large uvula or an enlarged base of the tongue that crowds the back of the throat may also cause sleep apnea. A jawbone or mandible that is short or displaced backward may cause the tongue to intrude on the back of the throat and decrease airflow. About two-thirds of the people with sleep apnea are overweight. For these, the accumulation of fat in the abdomen, neck, and throat may cause changes in breathing patterns, predisposed to blockage and decreasing airflow through the upper airway.

Examination of these areas by a physician can give clues as to whether you have obstructive sleep apnea. Some people with hypothyroidism have sleep apnea because of being overweight or because of changes in their control of ventilation by the central nervous system due to the low levels of the thyroid hormone. Interestingly, the incidence of sleep apnea in premenopausal women is much less than in men. For postmenopausal women, the incidence of sleep apnea approaches that of men. This happens because the location of fat deposits around the upper airway is similar in men and postmenopausal women. Also, those who take anabolic steroids such as testosterone have an increased chance of developing obstructive sleep apnea.

Diagnosis and Treatment of Sleep Apnea

To clinch the diagnosis of obstructive sleep apnea, your doctor will recommend special sleep studies. Polysomnography can provide an important assessment of the occurrence of apneas, measures of oxygenation during sleep, and electrocardiographic abnormalities. These tests also measure the severity of sleep fragmentation such as arousals, sleep-stage shifts, or shortage of REM sleep. Other sleep disorders that may be contributing to the excessive daytime sleepiness may also be detected.

Polysomnography includes recording by electroencephalography, electrooculography, and electromyography (see page 189) for sleep staging. Airflow at your nose and mouth, respiratory effort signaled from monitors on the chest wall and abdomen, oxygen levels, and leg movements are also recorded. Your body position (supine, prone, side) and electrocardiogram are noted. A sleep study should include a sufficient amount of REM and NREM sleep.

The Epworth Sleepiness Scale

How likely are you to doze off or fall asleep in the following situations, as opposed to just feeling tired? This refers to your usual way of life in recent times. Even if you have not done some of these things recently, try to imagine how they would have affected you. Use the following scale to choose the most appropriate number for each situation.

Would never doze	0
Slight chance of dozing	1
Moderate chance of dozing	2
High chance of dozing	3

SITUATION	CHANCE OF DOZING
Sitting and reading	____
Watching television	____
Sitting, inactive in a public place (for example, in a theater or meeting)	____
Lying down to rest in the afternoon	____
Sitting and talking with someone	____
Sitting quietly after lunch without alcohol	____
In a car, while stopped for a few minutes in traffic	____

A *respiratory disturbance index* (RDI) may be calculated to assess the severity of abnormal respiratory events, based on their frequency. The RDI gives the number of abnormal respiratory events per hour of sleep.

If you have snoring but no evidence of other symptoms, overnight oximetry (oxygen level monitoring) during sleep in your home may be helpful as a screening tool. If the test shows a significant pattern of oxygen drops, a full polysomnogram may be warranted for a definitive diagnosis.

Once the diagnosis of obstructive sleep apnea has been confirmed, your doctor will make sure that you understand the health risks associated with this disorder. Problems such as an increased tendency to suffer from high blood pressure, abnormal heart rhythms, strokes, and heart attacks are all attributed to sleep apnea.

The excessive daytime sleepiness itself may cause major complications. Impairment of your alertness can cause accidents in your job or during travel. Your performance at the office or in social settings can suffer from daytime sleepiness. You need to comprehend the risks of this condition and also the effectiveness of the various treatment methods that are available. Also, the choice of therapy needs to be made based on the specific nature and severity of the sleep apnea in each case.

Although researchers have not found a uniformly effective and safe drug for treating obstructive sleep apnea, there are some medications that are useful in certain people. If you have an underactive thyroid (hypothyroidism), thyroid hormone replacement is clearly useful. For postmenopausal women, taking the hormone progesterone may be helpful. Antidepressant drugs have worked well for some people with mild obstructive sleep apnea. These agents decrease the amount of REM sleep, the sleep stage during which apneas tend to be more severe, and thus improve the sleep-related breathing disorder indirectly. These drugs may also work by stimulating the nerves that control the muscles responsible for keeping the upper airway open.

Protriptyline, which is nonsedating, is one of the best-studied antidepressants used for sleep apnea. It is used in a dose of 5 to 20 milligrams at bedtime. The drawbacks are the annoying side effects that increase as the dosage is raised. These include dry mouth, urinary hesitancy or frequency, and impotence.

If you have sleep apnea, be careful to avoid alcohol and drugs such as benzodiazepines (Xanax, Valium, and Restoril), which depress the central nervous system, relax the upper airway musculature, and may worsen sleep apnea.

Various devices designed to pull the tongue forward have been used, as well as devices that pull the jawbone forward. While these devices work, they may be uncomfortable and reduce the quality of your sleep.

Two decades ago the gold standard for treatment of obstructive sleep apnea was tracheostomy, but acceptance of this now is low because of cosmetic reasons and complications such as bleeding or infection. Occasionally this treatment is still used in an emergency situation.

Nasal continuous positive airway pressure (CPAP) is now the treatment of choice for obstructive sleep apnea. The nasal CPAP is a custom-fit mask placed over your nose in a tight-fitting seal. A flexible hose attaches this mask to a pump that quietly produces a positive pressure within your upper airway. This pressure serves as a "pneumatic splint" which prevents collapse of the oropharynx during sleep, thus eliminating apnea. Nasal CPAP also gets rid of your snoring—a definite benefit for other family members. The quality of your sleep will improve and your daytime energy will be much better. Some people find using nasal CPAP difficult and must seek help and support from their doctors.

Surgery

If you cannot use nasal CPAP, where do you turn? There are several surgical procedures available that may be helpful. The most widely performed operation is called uvulopalatopharyngoplasty (UPPP). This involves the removal of your tonsils if a tonsillectomy was not performed previously. The surgeon then reduces the size of your soft palate and decreases the obstruction in this upper part of your throat. If the obstruction is lower (at the base of the tongue), this procedure will not work. Other surgical procedures are used in those with problems related to the bony structures of the face. However, since surgery is associated with risks and complications, you should only consider it as a last resort if you have severe obstructive sleep apnea.

Getting Some Zzzzs

There are many options available so you can enjoy healing and restful sleep. No matter which type of respiratory problem you have, talk with your doctor or sleep disorders specialist about your specific concerns and seek appropriate medication or treatment.

Part 3

Mind over Breath

chapter 10

Stress, Emotion, and Breathing

Having lived with chronic allergy and asthma most of her childhood and adolescent years, twenty-two-year-old Vanessa described her repeated bouts of congestion, sticky mucus, wheezing, and gasping for breath as making her feel "lost, overwhelmed, and beaten." Sadly, respiratory diseases had tainted her outlook on the future. Before she received the correct treatment to control the inflammation, these illnesses kept her from enjoying an active life as a young adult.

To feel "lost, overwhelmed, and beaten," as Vanessa described, is not difficult to understand when you consider what respiratory problems can do. Such symptoms as sneezing, runny nose, weepy eyes, and sore throat greet those with allergies on awakening. People with asthma and COPD feel the clutches of these breathtaking diseases throughout the day, as wheezing or coughing holds them back from doing the very activities that are normal and necessary, including being productive at work or enjoying their families. The chronic pain of sinusitis lingers with sufferers as they prepare for bedtime and even sends its nagging signals as they try to sleep. Chronic disease can drastically change people who are normally happy and free into people who are miserable and limited in all areas of life.

A Psychological Problem?

If your breathing problem has lasted for months or years, you may have sought psychological help because you were experiencing anxiety, fearfulness, depression, exhaustion, insomnia, irritability, or other problems. A chief barrier to overcoming this emotional grip occurs when well-meaning friends and family members suggest that the disease is "in your head." You have probably heard the following statements:

Maybe if you don't think about it (not breathing), it will go away.

You don't look like you're having trouble breathing. Are you sure it isn't something else?

Just put the allergy (asthma, sinusitis, COPD) out of your mind.

Maybe if you would move around more, you could breathe better.

Stop overreacting. You can catch your breath. You always did have a big imagination.

Since the medication isn't working, perhaps it is in your head.

Perhaps you should stop taking that medication the new doctor gave you. It is probably making the problem worse.

If you would quit worrying so much about your illness, maybe you would feel better.

After struggling day after day, year after year, with respiratory problems, you may even start to think that perhaps you are faking the illness or the problems are fabricated by your mind and emotions.

You must believe that the problems are *not* in your head; they are very real. Although studies have proven that emotional stress or worry can often exacerbate the breathing disorder, the problem is physical.

A chronic illness can take a tremendous emotional toll on the patient, and also on family and friends, but it is important to know that you are the same person—no matter what your symptoms may be. For example, instead of being tagged as an asthmatic, you need to see yourself as a normal person who happens to have asthma. Rather than being labeled as an allergic person, seeing yourself as a normal person who has allergies is vital.

To view yourself as normal and healthy in the midst of your breathing problem is a positive and accurate way to live. Clearly, the breathing disorder is uncomfortable and even frightening at times. However, you must focus on the things you do have control over in life, including how you envision yourself and your overall health.

Chronic Disease and Depression

One of the greatest problems with any chronic disease is that sufferers can become depressed and withdrawn. With breathing disorders, patients become ever more focused on their inability to breathe normally and on their personal suffering. The many appointments with physicians to try to find relief, combined with the cost of these attempts and the episodes of breathing difficulties, add to this frustration.

As time goes on, those who suffer with unmanaged asthma, allergy, COPD, or other chronic breathing problems can have trouble keeping a job; the absences become too frequent. If income is reduced or lost altogether, this adds to the financial stress for the patients and their families. The stress of dealing with loss of income, along with the breathing disorders, can cause relationship problems with loved ones and friends.

The longer breathing disorders go uncontrolled, the more likely the person will experience feelings and notice signs caused by the stress. This can make it more difficult to breathe and create even further problems, including:

Difficulty sleeping leading to constant fatigue

Inability to exercise leading to poor aerobic and physical fitness

Difficulty concentrating from the side effects of medications leading to poor performance

Increased irritability from lack of sleep or medications' side effects

Withdrawal from favorite activities because of low energy

Changes in appetite due to medications

Depression

We do not deny that emotional stress can trigger a host of health-related problems, ranging from memory loss to impaired immunity; it definitely plays a role in respiratory problems. However, thanks to extensive research, scientists have a better understanding of how stress affects the body. The fact is, stress is simply the trigger. Whether there will be health consequences following exposure to a stressful episode depends on your responses to the external event. These responses involve the immune system, heart and blood vessels, and certain glands that secrete hormones that help regulate various functions in the body, such as brain function and nerve impulses. All these responses interact and are profoundly influenced by one's coping style and psychological state. In short, stress does not cause respiratory problems but may worsen them. You can modify these internal responses as you practice the alternative or complementary mind-body exercises outlined in Chapter 11.

The Biology of Stress

"Stress is nothing new to me," you might say. "I live with it daily and have suffered its consequences." Yes, stress is here to stay. However, no two people respond in the same way to all stressful events. What may be a source of emotional excitement for you may be a form of abject terror for your best friend. People perceive and respond to stressors in different ways, but again, the negative responses adversely influence your health.

The Austrian physiologist Hans Selye introduced the general adaptation syndrome, which involves the biological changes that occur in response to a stressor which are beneficial as they enable you to adapt to the situation. This adaptation involves drawing on resources within the body to provide the energy and oxygen that your body needs to either *fight* or *flee*.

Try to think of this process as being like your savings account at the bank. You set funds aside for use in an emergency. When your car unexpectedly breaks down, your life is barely interrupted because you can afford to have it quickly repaired. The emergency will not severely affect your lifestyle because you have the money to deal with it.

Your body's currency is stored away as triglycerides and glycoproteins. The currency itself is glucose, along with amino and fatty acids. This is what fuels your brain as well as the muscles and other organ systems within your body. Without it, your body would literally shut down.

One of the first things that happens when you find yourself in a threatening situation is the activation of a pair of tiny glands in the body called the *adrenals*. They are controlled by cells in the brain, and their primary mission is to produce a chemical, or hormone, that converts stored energy into usable energy. We call this chemical *cortisol*. Without this chemical, you could not possibly survive an emergency. Cortisol puts energy in your personal tank in the form of blood glucose.

Now this source of energy is effective provided the emergency lasts only a short time. In biological terms, a short time would be a few hours, perhaps even a couple of days. Yet if the emergency lingers for weeks or months, problems arise. One of these problems is you are constantly withdrawing savings without replacing them. You use up all your body's resources until you reach a point when there are no more available. Then instead of drawing on naturally stored energy, the body begins breaking down muscle and other tissues to keep going.

Not just nonessential functions such as reproduction are shut down, but processes that are essential to long-term survival become impaired. This is because the same chemicals that help to mobilize resources within the body are also capable of impairing certain systems. For example, elevated levels of cortisol for extended periods of time will inhibit the ability of white cells to combat viral and other types of infections. When memory centers within the brain become bathed in high levels of cortisol, it becomes more difficult to encode information into memory. If the autonomic nervous system, which controls various functions such as heart rate, blood pressure, intestinal movement, and bronchial tube caliber, gets out of balance, problems within the cardiovascular, gastrointestinal, and pulmonary systems may very well occur. In short, the general adaptation syndrome evolved to take care of short-term emergencies. It was never intended to remain activated for extended periods of time.

Stress and Tuberculosis

It is important to understand that pulmonary problems can be triggered by emotional distress. For example, tuberculosis (see pages 282–85) results from a combination of exposure to the mycobacteria that trigger the specific symptoms, a genetic predisposition, and stress. Unlike HIV, tuberculosis is very easily transmitted, simply by inhaling the expired air of someone who has an active form of the disease.

Interestingly, not all people who are exposed come down with the disease. You might be standing with a friend on the same crowded bus when someone behind you suddenly coughs. Eventually your friend comes down with full-blown tuberculosis while you aren't even aware that you were exposed. In your body, the bacteria enters the lung where it becomes encapsulated in what is known as a *granuloma*. It becomes encased within this cellular prison and is unable to cause any health-related problems. Why the different responses?

Dr. Bruce Zwilling, a scientist at the Ohio State University School of Medicine, has been unraveling the mystery. His research with laboratory models reveals that some individuals are more likely to get certain types of infections than other individuals. These include infections by the special type of bacteria that causes tuberculosis.

Because the immune system is extremely complex, there is no question that some people are more susceptible to certain types of infections or problems such as allergy or asthma. Other people are less susceptible to those disorders but more vulnerable to others. Still, just because you have a genetic susceptibility to the tuberculosis bacteria does not result in the disease. There has to be *exposure* to the bacteria. Furthermore, in the models that Dr. Zwilling works with, the animals have to be exposed to a mild stressor as well. In other words, it is a combination of *stress, genetics,* and *exposure* that results in the disease.

Stress + genetics + exposure = disease

Weakened by Stress

How can stress influence the likelihood of developing tuberculosis or other chronic respiratory diseases? If stress weakens your immune system, you will be more likely to develop an illness. These illnesses include infections caused by the viruses that trigger common cold symptoms or herpes, fungi, and certain bacteria. We are frequently exposed to them, and often our bodies get rid of the infectious agent before it causes symptoms. That is because certain white blood cells mobilize immediately, wrap their membrane around the infectious agent, and destroy it when it enters the body.

Encounters such as this occur all the time. You develop what is called a subclinical infection. It is only when this first line of defense breaks down that the infectious agent can proliferate to the extent that it can trigger overt symptoms.

If you could take steps to ensure that your immune system was always alert and strong, you could avoid getting these infections. Unfortunately, there are many factors that can impair the ability of the defending white cells to do their job properly.

Controllable Factors That Impair Immune Function
Poor nutrition
Lack of sleep
Lack of exercise
Consumption of certain drugs
Stress, especially long-term

It is interesting that an increase of respiratory problems in young children has been strongly associated with starting primary school. This is undoubtedly related to the many infectious agents to which the children are exposed on entering school. It may also be related to the observation that salivary cortisol is significantly increased during the week before beginning kindergarten and for the first week of starting school. It has been suggested that children showing the greatest increase in cortisol due to the stress of starting school will have higher respiratory illness incidences in the weeks following the start of school. If you have a child, you may have experienced the relationship of starting school and a respiratory problem.

Chronic stress persists for weeks or even months. It is true that the immune system needs a certain amount of cortisol, which is the body's main stress-induced hormone. But when cortisol becomes extremely elevated as with chronic stress and remains so for an extended period of time, it can inhibit the lymphocytes, or white blood cells. Other chemicals produced by the brain's autopilot—known as the autonomic nervous system—can similarly damage the cells that make up the immune system.

During stress, you activate cortisol and the autonomic nervous system. Because of being bathed in the stress-related chemicals, the immune system may not keep infections in the subclinical phase. The virus or bacteria proliferate to the point where they infect many cells; this eventually leads to symptoms. The only way to get rid of the invader is to mobilize the second line of defense, which would include specialized white blood cells called the T cells and B cells.

During this time, cortisol may affect the number and function of these cells. While this is happening, you may suffer from a sore throat, runny nose, and itchy eyes if the encounter happened to be with some rhinovirus.

You need to know that stress did not cause your cold. The rhinovirus caused the cold. Exposure to that virus might not have resulted in problems if your immune system were working adequately. Because of your response to the stressor, your immune system was not working at full capacity. The role of stress in this scenario was to make it easier for the virus to cause the illness.

Immunologic Balance and Psychological Response

Whether you suffer with respiratory disease or not, you need to seek immunologic balance. The stress hormone cortisol helps you to achieve that balance. Because cortisol is intimately regulated by the so-called limbic, or emotional, brain, emotional stress can, through this hormone, have a profound impact on the immune system.

As often happens when talking about issues related to health, it is not nearly as simple as you might think. While there are people who are vulnerable to infections and other people who are susceptible to inflammatory disease, the majority of people have no changes in their immune system at all in response to a stressor.

First, during stress there are many hormones produced by the body, including some that augment the immune system. The latter would include prolactin and growth hormones. Whether the immune system is going to be affected is determined in large part not by the concentration of any one hormone but instead by the relative amounts of several different ones. Furthermore, these hormones are profoundly influenced by a person's psychological responses.

Perception

Of the four psychological responses, perception is absolutely paramount. Unless you think that something is going to be a threat, it is not going to trigger the so-called alarm phase of the general adaptation syndrome. This is the initial stage of the stress response, when you realize that there is a potential threat to your well-being.

Your best friend may look forward to going to the airport on her day off and jumping out of a perfectly functional airplane as a member of a skydiving club. For her, this is a positive experience and constitutes a form of emotional excitement. Nevertheless, you may respond to even the sound of airplanes taking off and landing with great anxiety. While the environmental trigger—the airplane—is identical, different people perceive the situation in totally different ways.

Different individuals also have different susceptibilities to stress. We all need a certain amount of emotional excitement in our lives to counter the effects of boredom and tedium. You may achieve all the emotional excitement you need by reading a Stephen King novel or watching a suspenseful video in your home. A friend of yours may have a very high threshold for emotional excitement and achieve it by jumping off cranes with bungee cords around her ankles or by participating in other dangerous sports. Your threshold for responding to stress is dictated largely by your genetic blueprint.

Control

When you perceive that you no longer are in control, emotional excitement, which is positive, turns into anxiety, which is negative. There is a very fine line between the two conditions. It is similar to the fence that might separate you from a caged lion at the zoo. The same animal 10 feet from where you are standing is simply an object of curiosity when there is a protective barrier. The moment that barrier is removed, that animal becomes a threat. Being in control is similar to that protective barrier. When the sense of control is lost and you feel helpless, anxiety and subsequent health problems will occur.

Coping Style

Coping style is another psychological variable that can influence your health. You probably know people who are always tense. The slightest aggravation causes them to go off the deep end. Their heart rate may soar, and they may perspire profusely with the slightest aggravation. Their pattern of breathing may become rapid and shallow.

In patients with underlying lung disease, the arterial blood gases may become very abnormal and cause problems such as dizziness or lethargy. Interestingly, shortness of breath without a change in respiratory rate or depth may be a symptom of anxiety. In some people, frequent sighing may be a sign of this as well. Not only that but when these individuals fill out psychological questionnaires, they say that they are highly anxious. This is the category to which they belong.

Then there are people who are at the opposite end of the spectrum. They are referred to as low anxious. You practically have to light a stick of dynamite under them to get any response at all.

Naturally, there is still another group that can be found midway between these two. These are individuals who react the same way that highly anxious people do but, when asked about their method of coping, claim that they are low anxious. These are people who repress their feelings. These are also individuals who are more prone to infections and more likely to have a worse course when dealing with cancer.

Personality Type

Finally, personality type can have a profound impact on susceptibility to illness. You have probably heard of the so-

called Type A personality. These individuals are quite literally slaves to the clock. They are always in a hurry and sel-
dom take time out to enjoy life. They are time oriented and
frequently speak with a very rapid rate of speech, finishing
the sentences of those they are speaking to as they grow
impatient. This is in marked contrast to the Type B personality who is quite simply a non-Type A. Type B people get
the work done but also take time out to smell the roses.

It was initially concluded that it was the Type A individual who was most likely to succumb to a heart attack. That
conclusion is still to be found in many basic psychology
textbooks. That is only partly true, however. We now know
that it is not so much the time orientation that is responsible for the associated heart problems but more the emotions associated with stress. Anger and hostility account for
the correlation between the Type A personality and heart
disease. In other words, it is probably okay to be a workaholic; just don't be an angry, hostile workaholic!

The Type C personality has been correlated with certain forms of cancer. This individual is strikingly similar to
the so-called rheumatoid arthritic personality, a term
coined by Dr. George Solomon in the mid-1960s. Both
personalities are extremely passive and are willing to
endure a great deal of personal discomfort to please other
people. It is the person who will frequently say yes when
he or she really wants to say no. There may be many reasons why this individual is more vulnerable to infections
and certain forms of cancer, but one may be related to the
issue of control.

In a sense, people who allow their actions to be dictated by others are not in control of their lives. In extreme
cases, they form codependent relationships with others
that can be extremely unhealthy for both members of the
relationship.

A final type personality is the so-called Type T, or thrill-seeking, personality. There are no classic diseases associated with taking risks that we are aware of, although these individuals do have a decreased life expectancy because of the risks that they do take. It is noteworthy, however, that most drug addicts are Type T personalities. That does not mean that most Type Ts are drug addicts, simply that most addicts enjoy taking risks. This fits with the hypothesis of many mental health workers that many addicts are addicted not only to the chemical formulations that they abuse but also to the risk associated with living on the edge. They become addicted to the thrill associated with stealing to support their habit or perhaps even the risk associated with the changes in their health.

The categorization of people into discrete personality types is useful as a model from a purely experimental standpoint, but it is not an exact depiction of reality. There is no such thing as a "pure" Type A, B, C, or T personality. Although it is true that our genetic code and early experiences can have a profound impact on our ultimate personality, the environment in which we find ourselves is equally important. There is a certain amount of overlap among the various model personalities. For example, you may be a classic Type A personality at work, a Type B at home with your family, and then a Type C when you check into the hospital.

In other words, you may be a composite of all these personalities. It does turn out, though, that most of the time you will exhibit the characteristics of one or just a couple of these personality constructs.

While this is a useful way to categorize people, it might be more accurate to think of personalities as coping styles that enable people to deal with problems in their immediate environment. These are just a few of the many factors that can affect the immune system, especially the way that it responds to stressors.

Stress and Allergy

While perception, sense of control, coping skills, and personality types are the major psychological factors that can impact your immune system and its response to stressors, there is still another important factor—the *autonomic nervous system*. This part of the nervous system has two branches, the *sympathetic* and *parasympathetic*, which work with each other to control some involuntary activities of the body. Excessive levels of *epinephrine*, the main chemical produced by the sympathetic branch, can suppress many parts of the immune system. Since an allergic reaction is an overzealous immune response to animal dander, pollen, or another allergen, then you might think of epinephrine in this context as beneficial. For example, epinephrine is a bronchodilator. That is precisely why doctors inject patients with epinephrine when they are in danger of going into anaphylactic shock, as discussed on page 24. This is the same epinephrine that the adrenal gland would normally produce in response to signals from the autonomic nervous system, but now a little extra is administered to help ward off potentially lethal problems.

On the other hand, *acetylcholine,* which is produced by the parasympathetic branch of the autonomic nervous system, can do just the opposite. It can stimulate the release of histamine, serotonin, and other chemical mediators from mast cells and basophils, a type of white blood cell that releases chemicals that can cause bronchoconstriction. As you now know from earlier sections of this book, agents such as histamine cause bronchoconstrictions and mucus secretions that are detrimental to bronchial tube or nasal function. Acetylcholine then is not the chemical you want circulating in the body in large amounts during an allergic reaction! Atropine or an atropine-like substance such as ipratropium (see page 106), which is in the medication Atrovent, is sometimes useful because it blocks the effects of acetylcholine. Ask your doctor if this medication may help your situation.

Individuals have discovered that emotional distress has an immediate impact on their allergic symptoms. For some, stress makes their symptoms get better, whereas for others it makes them get worse. There may be many reasons for this, but one is a possible imbalance within the autonomic nervous system. For example, some people may produce more epinephrine under stress, and thereby alleviate their symptoms. Other people produce more acetylcholine and have a worsening of their symptoms. Research has shown that psychological factors can interact with asthma to worsen or improve the disease through alterations in the autonomic system.

Behavioral Interventions

Although severe emotional stress can cause an imbalance, you have many options at your disposal, as suggested throughout this book, to reestablish harmony within your immune system, as well as a host of other physiological systems. Without question, the chemicals produced during moderate exercise can be extremely beneficial in enhancing the function of the immune system. Regular aerobic and strengthening exercise is also a very effective way to train your body to deal with stress under controlled circumstances. And, of course, volumes have been written about the health benefits of nutrition. We are indeed what we eat from an immunologic standpoint, as well. Nearly all the immune system cells benefit from a varied and well-balanced diet. Without adequate amounts of vitamins such as C and beta-carotene the immune system will malfunction. Music, humor, aromatherapy, deep abdominal breathing, massage, and faith, as outlined in Chapter 11, are other ways that people have found effective in maintaining a state of good health.

One of the most effective interventions which costs very little money if any at all is social support. For example, there is no question that loneliness is as much a risk factor for disease as high cholesterol or smoking cigarettes. It is well documented that people who are happily married or have large networks of friends not only have greater life expectancies compared with those people who do not, but they also have fewer incidences of just about all types of disease. Dr. David Spiegel is a psychiatrist at Stanford University who documented what many scientists had speculated about: Social support can be a significant factor in prolonging the lives of women with breast cancer. This simple intervention prolonged life expectancy by an average of eighteen months.

However, social support does not have to be just in relationships with other people. You may form emotional attachments with your animals. This is every bit as strong as the attachment between a parent and a child. There are countless papers published in the area of animal-human bonding revealing the health benefits of this type interaction. Even having a plant can be beneficial. This was revealed in a study conducted at Yale University by Dr. Judy Rhodin who found that when people had a plant present in their room, they had speedier recoveries compared with people who did not. The common denominator among all these studies is the word responsibility—responsibility for a loved one, a pet, and even a plant. Taking this idea one step further, one could argue that accepting responsibility for one's own health is by itself a behavioral intervention that is conducive to recovery.

The Role of Psychotherapy

Most people with chronic respiratory diseases live with unending stress. This stress makes it more difficult to handle everyday issues, much less crises that may arise. One woman who had lived with uncontrolled allergies for years described her personality as Dr. Jekyll and Mr. Hyde, warning friends to stay away on days her illness flared.

Once you accept that your emotional status can affect both your perception of your illness as well as your ability to develop appropriate coping strategies, you can make positive changes. The role of psychological counseling in a management program can help you develop appropriate coping strategies to deal with these issues. Psychological intervention is an accepted component for everyone, not just people who have "psychological problems." Psychological intervention can give you coping methods that you can use either within or outside other treatment programs. In most cases, it is important that the person providing these services is familiar with respiratory problems. Some of these methods include the following.

Individual Counseling

This is a one-on-one session with a therapist in which individual problem areas are addressed. These sessions may include specific help alleviating depression, anxiety, or stress, along with other personal problem areas.

Family Counseling

Respiratory problems can extend beyond you and affect your entire family. Therefore, it is often helpful for family members to understand and accept your limitations and the possible impact they may have on your family's lifestyle. Family members can have the best of intentions, but without specific guidance, they sometimes make things worse. Family meetings may help you discuss the problems you have openly and get support to accomplish the activities of daily living.

Group Counseling

There is no one who can better understand you than another person with respiratory problems. Group sessions led by trained therapists allow sharing feelings, as well as developing effective coping strategies. The exchange of ideas at group sessions is often the most productive way to revamp your thought processes.

Support Groups

In a support group, you can share your feelings with others suffering from similar problems and receive comfort and encouragement from each other. The latest available treatments can be discussed and members can give coping suggestions while affirming the positive experiences of each other. The realization that "someone else knows what I am going through" is helpful as people share their struggle in living with breathing disorders.

Support groups are not meant to be professional therapy groups. Those who would benefit from standard psychological or psychiatric intervention should seek professional treatment to fit their needs.

Finding workable answers is important as you seek to change your emotional response. A host of alternative intervention strategies are presented in the following chapter. No matter which choices you make and carry out in your lifestyle, accepting responsibility for your health and your quality of life is of paramount importance.

chapter 11

Alternative Treatments: Mind-Body Healing

Although traditional medical treatments afford many lifesaving and life-extending therapies, especially with the newer inhaled and preventive medications, millions of people have found additional improvement with a complementary or holistic approach, including relaxation, biofeedback, nutritional foods, exercise, and herbs. For example, yoga breathing exercises or Chinese tai chi encourages relaxed breathing and panic control. Modern biofeedback may help in treating panic or anxiety attacks, especially important for those who fear the next attack of wheezing or shortness of breath. The importance of nutritional foods has been stressed earlier in the book (see "Antioxidants," pages 164 to 171, and "Elimination Diets," pages 162–64). Therapeutic massage (TM) has been used for decades to loosen the phlegm that accompanies asthma, bronchitis, and COPD. Deep abdominal breathing helps to reduce stress symptoms and the detrimental effect on the respiratory system. Likewise, music therapy provides relaxation for many and helps to lower a racing heart rate.

Caution

A common mistake made by many when they use alternative medicine practitioners (both physician and nonphysician) is that they stop the traditional medical treatment altogether. This one mistake can often lead to life-threatening respiratory episodes or setbacks. It is important to continue your regular medical therapy and have your physician's approval before complementing your management plan with any alternative therapy.

Stress and Airway Constriction

As discussed in Chapter 10, a negative response to emotional stress has a powerful influence on victims of many types of breathing disorders. On the basis of scientific tests, we know that the emotion or worry causes the body to produce the chemical acetylcholine, which causes the airways to constrict. When enough acetylcholine is secreted, the result may be asthma.

In one study, researchers told a group of asthmatics that they were being exposed to pollens and other aggravating triggers. Then the researchers stood back and watched what happened. More than half of the asthmatics developed a full-blown asthma attack, although no pollens or other substances were present. Worry that it might happen triggered a very real attack. The power of suggestion is that strong.

If you have trouble breathing, it is important to learn how to control worry and negative responses to stressors. Let's look at some of the most common forms of alternative or complementary treatments that can help you to stay in control.

Relaxation Response

The relaxation response, first described by Dr. Herbert Benson more than twenty years ago, is one of the most-studied methods to reduce stress and benefit those with respiratory problems. Recent studies have found that relaxation therapy appears to produce improved adjustment, increased medication compliance, and decreased use of medical services for those with respiratory disorders.

The stress of having chronic breathing problems or even worrying about having shortness of breath can put you into emotional overload. Breathing problems can affect your mood and cause irritability, impatience, and higher levels of frustration. However, although breathing problems are considered a physical problem, as we discussed in Chapter 10 emotional fears and other stress factors play an overall role in the experience. For example, think of a time when you cut your finger but did not have pain until you looked at the finger and saw blood. Likewise, just the anticipation or fear of not breathing well, even if there is not an immediate problem, can cause an increase in your heart rate and quickening in your breathing which makes the respiratory system do even more work.

Relaxation can offer a potential to reduce physical strain and emotional, negative thoughts and increase your ability to self-manage stress. Each of these benefits has a positive effect on your illness.

To begin your own stress reduction program, set aside a period of about twenty minutes each day that you can devote to relaxation practice. As much as possible, remove outside distractions that can disrupt your concentration: turn off the radio, the television, even the ringer on the telephone if necessary. During practice, it is important to recline comfortably so that your whole body is supported and as much tension or tightness in your muscles is relieved as possible. This is difficult to do upright, since your muscles must be tightened to maintain the position.

You can use a pillow or cushion under your head if this helps.

During the twenty-minute period, remain as still as you can. Focus your thoughts as much as possible on the immediate moment, and eliminate any outside thoughts which may compete for your attention. Try to notice which parts of your body feel relaxed and loose and which parts feel tense and uptight.

As you go through these steps, in your own way try to imagine that every muscle in your body is becoming loose, relaxed, and free of any excess tension. Picture all the muscles in your body beginning to unwind; imagine them beginning to go loose and limp. Concentrate on making your breathing slow, even, and rhythmic. As you exhale on each breath, picture your muscles becoming even more relaxed, as if with each breath you breathe the tension away. At the end of twenty minutes, take a few moments to study and focus on the feelings and sensations you have been able to achieve. Notice whether areas that felt tight and tense at first now feel more loose and relaxed and whether any areas of tension or tightness remain.

Don't be surprised if the relaxed feeling you achieved begins to fade and dissipate once you get up and return to your normal activities. Many people find that it is only after several weeks of daily practice that they are able to maintain the relaxed feeling beyond the practice session itself.

If you practice regularly, your body will soon learn to elicit the relaxation response and target the sympathetic nervous system. This, in turn, will help relieve the anxiety and reduce the adrenaline that often accompanies shortness of breath. For professional instruction on relaxation, seeing a clinical psychologist who specializes in working with these problems may be beneficial.

Deep Abdominal Breathing

Breathing can measure and alter your psychological state, making a stressful moment accelerate or diminish in intensity. Think about how your respiration quickens when you are fearful or in great pain and how taking a deep, slow breath can be calming and reduce both stress and levels of muscle pain. But how often we take breathing for granted. This is one of the few activities of the body that we can consciously control. As you learn how to do deep abdominal breathing, you will gain control over a basic physiological function; this will help decrease the release of stress hormones and slow down your heart rate during stressful moments. Also, by adding oxygen to the blood, you can cause your body to release endorphins—the "happy" hormones that give a greater sense of well-being and contentment.

Lie on your back in a quiet room with no distractions. If necessary, take the phone off the hook. Place your hands on your abdomen, and take in a slow, deliberate deep breath through your nostrils. If your hands are rising and your abdomen is expanding, then you are breathing correctly. If your hands do not rise and you see your chest rising, you are breathing incorrectly.

Inhale to a count of five, pause for three seconds, then exhale to a count of five. Start with ten repetitions of this exercise, and then increase to twenty-five, twice daily. Use this exercise any time you feel anxious or stressed.

You might find this exercise extremely helpful when you are experiencing chest tightness from tension and anxiety. The slow, deep breathing can interrupt a cycle of rapid, shallow breathing and result in less distortion of oxygen and carbon dioxide in the blood, as well as a more comfortable state of mind.

Progressive Muscle Relaxation

Progressive muscle relaxation involves contracting and then relaxing all the different muscle groups in the body, beginning with your head and neck and progressing down to your arms, chest, back, stomach, pelvis, legs, and feet. To do this exercise, you focus on each set of muscles, tense these muscles to the count of ten, and then release to the count of ten. Go slowly as you progress throughout your entire body; take as long as you can. Get in touch with each part and feel the tension you are experiencing. Also, notice how it feels to be tension-free as you release the muscle.

Studies show that when you can create a restful mental image using this type of relaxation technique, you feel removed from cumbersome stress and negative emotions. This mindfulness, or focusing all attention of what you feel from moment to moment, can also help you move beyond destructive habits as you become centered in a world of health and inner healing.

You can do progressive muscle relaxation with or without music, and it is important to do it with deep abdominal breathing, focusing on your breath. Breathe in while tensing the muscles; breathe out while relaxing them.

Visualization, or Guided Imagery

Visualization, or guided imagery, has been used successfully for controlling emotional distress, anxiety, and depression in chronically ill people. This simple, inexpensive technique is one that we all have the potential to master. Studies on those with COPD suggest that guided imagery may even significantly improve one's perceived quality of life.

Granted, some people are naturally better at imaging than others, but we can all learn to visualize effectively if we practice. Much like learning to play the piano or tennis, becoming skilled at guided imagery involves time, patience, and practice. This is a skill that cannot be rushed or hurried.

To practice guided imagery, you need to be alone in a quiet environment without distractions. During this time-out, try to visualize a peaceful, relaxing scene, perhaps a vacation spot you have enjoyed in the mountains or at the seashore. Whatever the scene is, focus on this place. Try to recapture the moment as you imagine the sounds, smells, textures, and feelings of being at this place. Become more aware of your breathing and anxiety level as you continue your focus, and do not let outside stimuli hinder your imagery time.

Through guided imagery, you can reduce your anxiety level during stressful times and even lower your heart rate and blood pressure. As you continually visualize a positive healing image, you may significantly contribute to your own well-being.

Music Therapy

Music therapy is an effective approach to help in reducing fear, anxiety, stress, or grief. It is just beginning to make its mark as a way to reduce the stress that accompanies respiratory problems. In one study 106 asthmatic subjects were medically prestabilized and then exposed to eight sessions of progressive relaxation, music, or waiting without any therapy. Listening to music produced greater decreases in peaks of tension than progressive relaxation, and it produced greater compliance with relaxation practice.

If you use music to unwind, avoid melodies that make you tense or that cause uneasiness. Spend ten to twenty minutes a day listening to music, and try this in combination with another mind-body technique, such as guided imagery, deep abdominal breathing, or progressive muscle relaxation. Make sure that the pace of the music you choose is slower than your heart rate, or approximately sixty beats a minute. This rhythm encourages your heart rate to slow down. Some studies of late have shown that this will also lower blood pressure and could boost your immune function while reducing your levels of stress hormones.

Aromatherapy

At this time research is being conducted on aromas or scents and how they may alter people's moods. Some studies have been done on the inhalation of scents, yet the term aromatherapy extends far beyond this to include the use of certain oils. Each of the different oils is suggested to have a specific healing power, whether to reduce stress, fight infection, increase energy, or serve as an aphrodisiac. For example, lavender and spiced apples are said to increase the alpha wave activity in the back of the brain; this leads to relaxation. Conversely, increased beta activity in the front of the brain shows greater alertness and is said to occur with the smell of jasmine or lemon. Some research has found chamomile oil to be an anti-inflammatory and clove oil to be antimicrobial.

Revealing studies performed in Japan reported that when certain scents were delivered through the air-conditioning ducts, the workers displayed increased efficiency and lower stress. Jasmine was found to decrease the rate of errors per hour by 33 percent. This rate of errors dropped by an astounding 53 percent when the fragrance of lemon was emitted. Workers also had a more positive sense of well-being during this time.

It is probably no news that certain scents such as eucalyptus help open mucous membranes or at least make you feel as if you can breathe better. Perhaps this is why eucalyptus over-the-counter cough drops and chest rubs have been popular with many for generations. Studies have shown that eucalyptus is an essential oil used by cultures around the world for treating diseases involving the respiratory system. Breathing the steam of peppermint essential oil is also used by some as a decongestant, destressor, and aid to ease sinus headache pain.

Does aromatherapy work? Although there have been no controlled studies to date, some say they feel better when using aromatherapy. Whether aromas can reduce the stress of chronic breathing problems depends on each person's response. Keep in mind that aromatherapy is one alternative treatment that must be approached with great caution. Aromas and fumes may act as major triggers for millions with allergy and asthma and can even be life threatening.

A Merry Heart

While the finding is disheartening, it may come as no surprise that the average adult only laughs about 17 times a day, whereas a six-year-old laughs as many as 300 times. Although laughter cannot make your wheezing or sneezing banish, it can make it easier to live with a chronic illness. Simply stated, humor helps to relieve anxiety and allows you to regain a healthy outlook on life. Hospitals across the country are using this form of laughter therapy by providing patients with humor rooms and comedy carts.

Norman Cousins was the first to promote laughter as an antidote to disease. When Cousins was the editor of the *Saturday Review,* he was diagnosed with a serious connective tissue disease. Although his doctors said that it was incurable, he was determined to get well.

During his journey to find a cure for his ailment,

Cousins discovered that positive thoughts and genuine laughter affected his body chemistry for the better. He filled his life with movies that made him laugh—a real belly laugh. He then documented his account of the "miraculous recovery by laughter," in the book *Anatomy of an Illness as Perceived by the Patient*. As he recovered from his "incurable" illness, Cousins went on to tell others of the miracle power of laughter and the positive chemical changes in the body.

There is a growing body of evidence that supports what Cousins experienced. This research links laughter and a strengthened immune system with an increase in T cells, as well as natural killer (NK) cell activity. The T cells attack cells infected by viruses or foreign cells to which the body has previously been exposed. Natural killer cells attack foreign cells, virus-infected cells, and cancer cells without prior exposure. Researchers have found that as little as twenty seconds of laughter can double the heart rate just like aerobic exercise; this makes it beneficial to the respiratory system, the central nervous system, and the cardiovascular system.

The only problem with laughing for good health is that for those with asthma or other chronic lung diseases, laughter can easily exacerbate the symptoms, that is, cause increased cough, wheeze, and inflammation. Just be sure to use your controller and reliever medications before you sit down with a comical magazine or a humorous video.

The Faith Factor

Researchers in the field of psychoneuroimmunology (mind-body interplay) report growing evidence on the positive effects of religion or faith on your health. These scientists contend that the human body has a powerful sacramental dimension to it, and those who acknowledge this with a strong sense of higher purpose—a body-soul connectedness—are the ones who are more likely to stay with programs that lead to optimal health. This does not mean that belief in God should ever replace medicine. However, knowing that faith in something greater than yourself offers a type of curative power that helps you to disconnect unhealthy worries and replace them with soothing belief.

In Greek, the word for faith is *pistis,* which means the act of giving one's trust. Trusting in God permits us to trust and commit to proven medical, nutritional, or fitness regimes we know will benefit us. Likewise, according to the latest medical research, faith in God is healthy and even healing. Many studies of late have found that people who are active in religious organizations and attend group functions regularly are healthier, with reports of lower blood pressure, less depression, and greater longevity.

This belief that your mind and spirit can have a dramatic effect on your physical body is not new. In the 2000-year-old Hippocratic writings, there are observations that "there is a measure of conscious thought throughout the body." Dr. Dean Ornish's successful program for reversing heart disease is based on a disciplined and meditative lifestyle that focuses on healing inner peace along with exercise and a healthful nutrition plan. Bill Moyers also confirmed the spiritual dimension of health in his groundbreaking PBS TV series and book, *Healing and the Mind.* Moyers found that there is, in fact, a relationship between our emotions and spiritual state and our bodies.

Many tell of using prayer and meditation to give comfort during episodes of dyspnea. The body switches from the pumping fight-or-flight response into a calmer mode during these spiritual disciplines. Studies show that prayer and meditation produce alpha and theta waves consistent with serenity and happiness, and so allow your harried thoughts to have a reprive.

Groundbreaking research is revealing that these disciplines can also literally reconfigure the brain biology and trigger biochemical and neurological changes that are therapeutic. This reconfiguring can make a big difference in one's health and well-being. Just as scientists have found that positive beliefs can engender wellness (the placebo effect), they also have found that negative beliefs and influences can induce illness (the "nocebo" effect), as with the asthmatics who were told they were exposed to pollen but were not (see page 229).

One woman said that prayer helped her to relax when she felt her chest tightening from asthma; this made it easier for her to catch her breath. A young man with chronic sinusitis and asthma who practices meditation twice daily said this helps him to focus on breathing correctly and gives him hope for healing. Prayer and meditation provide nourishment for your soul, satiate that inner spiritual hunger, and help you develop your ability to pay attention to all areas of your life without distraction.

There is no proof that these mind-body tools cause healing. However, there are more studies showing that those who find strength and comfort in their religion have better survival rates from serious disease as well as a higher quality of life than those who claim to be nonreligious.

Ancient Disciplines for Relaxation

Chi gong ho

This ancient Chinese art of self-healing consists of a series of breathing and moving exercises and has helped millions for more than 5,000 years reduce pain and increase mobility when no other exercise has worked. *Chi* (meaning "energy") and *gong* (meaning "cultivation") has been said to induce the relaxation response in those who practice it regularly. Chi gong ho is based on the belief that a powerful energy system called chi circulates through the body and regulates the body's organic functions. Chi oxygenates the blood and nourishes the organs; it surrounds the body as an aura.

Many community colleges, YMCAs, and private schools offer courses in chi gong ho. However, make sure that a certified instructor teaches the course you take.

Tai chi

Tai chi may give an added benefit especially to elderly people in warding off age-related breathing problems. In a study reported in the *Journal of the American Geriatrics Society* (1995), tai chi was found to help improve lung function in older people. Sometimes endurance exercises are too taxing for older people. This ancient discipline with its deep-breathing component may help people to maintain better lung function. Other studies have shown those senior adults who regularly did this exercise experienced greater spinal flexibility and increased ability to take in oxygen than those who did not.

With tai chi, you follow a series of slow, graceful movements that mimic the movements you do in daily life. You move forward, backward, and from side to side in a carefully, coordinated manner—flowing together as though your body was doing one continuous movement.

Since the exercise emphasizes complete relaxation and passive concentration, it can be characterized as meditation in motion. Tai chi is said to speed healing, improve circulation, boost immune function, and decrease stress.

Dramatic, flowing movements are used instead of forceful actions. The exercise emphasizes deep abdominal breathing that could help to maintain better lung function. As a low-impact exercise, it is perfect for older people or those who have severe breathing difficulties. It increases the heart rate and helps to improve overall cardiovascular function.

There are books on tai chi along with videos that you can purchase and use in the privacy of your home. Or, you may enjoy the company of doing this with others at a local health spa or YMCA.

Yoga

Yoga may be helpful with some respiratory problems. It not only provides the benefit of relaxing your body, the various positions can help to improve your breathing and ease your expectoration of mucus.

Relaxation, flexibility, and muscle strength are important outcomes of yoga; this makes it a good exercise for those with chronic respiratory problems who are unable to do more aerobic-type exercises. With yoga, there is no high impact or bouncing.

Chiropractic

Chiropractic is a drug-free approach that relies on the manipulation of the spine and muscles, in conjunction with nutrition and exercise. Doctors of chiropractic are unique in that instead of treating the symptoms of a patient, they are primarily interested in treating the spinal bones when they are thought to lose their normal position and motion from stress, trauma, or other causes. Doctors of chiropractic are licensed by each state and must complete two years of undergraduate study, along with a four-year course at a chiropractic college.

How is it supposed to work? Your nervous system

controls all functions in your body; every cell in your body is supplied with nerve impulses. Messages must travel from your brain down your spinal cord, then out to the nerves at particular parts of the body, and then back to the spinal cord and back up the spinal cord to the brain. Chiropractic theory is that abnormal positions of the spinal bones may interfere with these messages and are often the underlying cause of many health problems.

Doctors of chiropractic correct the abnormal positions of the spinal bones with what is called an adjustment or manipulation. Either the doctor's hands or a specially designed instrument applies a brief and accurate thrust to a joint. Adjustments are said to help return the bones to a more normal position or motion, and so relieve pain and reduce ill health.

The chiropractic doctor may also recommend a program of rehabilitation for your spine. This phase of care is similar to orthodontics with the goal of stabilizing and reducing joint involvement, rehabilitating muscle, and balancing nerve impulses to help you regain maximum health. Many chiropractors feel that patients can see improvement in five to six visits and should be prepared to receive adjustments for at least one month. Patients who happen to get significant relief from spinal manipulation find that it helps them to continue with their management plan of prescribed medications such as preventer and reliever inhalers.

At this point, some discussion of the placebo response phenomenon is necessary. *Placebo* is Latin for "I shall please" (the opening phrase of the Catholic vespers for the dead to which the word ironically referred in its original context). Placebos are usually viewed as fake treatments like sugar pills that doctors give merely to please or calm anxious patients or to indulge insatiable ones. However, it has been shown that the placebo effect yields beneficial effects in 60 to 90 percent of diseases that include angina pectoris, bronchial asthma, herpes simplex, and duodenal ulcer. Three elements are involved in this effect:

1. Positive belief and expectations by the patient
2. Positive belief and expectations by the physician or health care provider
3. A good relationship between physician and patient.

Interestingly, some interventions that can be considered placebo, unreal, or inert turn out to produce various biochemical or physiologic changes. Some patients may have subjective improvement of asthma (symptoms) without objective improvement as in peak flow rates or spirometry. Although not everyone responds to placebos, it is reported that 30 to 40 percent of those treated responded to placebo and up to 55 percent responded in terms of pain relief. Unfortunately, there is no way to select a consistent placebo responder.

Whether chiropractic can be considered a placebo is not certain. One particular study from Copenhagen was a randomized patient- and observer-blinded crossover trial (well designed) which involved thirty-one patients ages eighteen to forty-four who suffered from chronic asthma. Their symptoms were controlled by bronchodilators or inhaled steroids. Patients were randomized to receive either active chiropractic spinal manipulation or sham manipulation twice weekly for four weeks. The patients then crossed over to the other treatment for another four weeks. Both phases were preceded and followed by a two-week period without chiropractic treatment. The main outcome measurements included FEV-1, amount of daily use of inhaled reliever bronchodilators, and nonspecific bronchial reactivity. No clinically important or statistically significant differences were found between the active and sham interventions on any of the main or secondary outcome measures, and objective lung function did not change during the study.

Massage and Therapeutic Touch

Studies released from the University of Miami School of Medicine's Touch Research Center found that the benefits of massage include heightened alertness, relief from depression and anxiety, an increase in the number of natural killer cells in the immune system, lower levels of the stress hormone cortisol, and reduced difficulty in getting to sleep. For those with respiratory conditions, therapeutic touch is frequently suggested to help patients increase their expectoration and relax their back, shoulder, neck, and chest musculature for enhanced breathing.

Therapeutic touch affects the body as a whole. This form of drugless therapy has been shown to increase circulation, give relief from musculoskeletal pain and tension, act as a mind-body form of stress release, increase flexibility, and increase mobility.

Several techniques used with success include:

General Swedish A full body massage with particular attention to back and chest

Vibration Anterior and posterior thoracic region coordinated with breath exhalation, the heel of the right hand used for vibration and the left hand placed on top of the right for light compression

Tapotement Anterior and posterior thoracic region, hand-edge hacking, cupping, and finger tapping with both hands

Trigger point Active and latent trigger points located and held with mild to moderate pressure for one to three minutes in the neck, shoulder, upper back, and chest

The American Massage Therapy Association provides a national referral service for qualified, professional massage therapists. Some licensed physical therapists and registered nurses now practice massage therapy as well.

Acupuncture

Acupuncture is a form of hyperstimulation for pain or symptom relief that has been approved by the Food and Drug Administration as a medical device. Researchers cannot explain how or why it works but have increasing evidence that there may be a physiological explanation for the therapy. This is significant because the types of drugs people with breathing disorders take can often cause nervousness or anxiety as a side effect. For example, beta2-agonists, a kind of drug prescribed to relax the muscles of the airways, and so make it easier to breathe, can cause headaches, anxiety, and tremors in some patients.

Relief from acupuncture is experienced through certain reflexes in the body that occur by way of the nervous system. That is to say, by stimulating one portion of the body and using pathways of the nervous system, an effect is obtained in the same or another portion of the body. Additionally, it is believed that acupuncture causes the body to release endorphins—the body's own pain-relieving chemicals; this may add to the feeling of relaxation. A hormone that fights inflammation is also produced in the body and may be triggered during acupuncture; this could explain why people with arthritis, migraine headache, and asthma have found relief with this type of alternative treatment. Some studies even suggest that acupuncture may trigger the release of certain neural hormones including serotonin, which adds to the feelings of calmness.

With acupuncture treatment fine-gauge sterilized needles are placed at various points selected by the practitioner. The needles are usually kept in place fifteen to thirty minutes. The doctor may periodically stimulate the needles by manually twisting them to obtain improved results.

Another form of stimulating the acupuncture points once the needle is in place is hooking up small wires connected to very slight electrical currents. This is known as electroacupuncture. Heat (moxibustion) and massage (acupressure) are also used during this process.

There are also ways of applying acupuncture today that do not require needles. Very sophisticated pieces of electronic equipment help the doctor detect the local acupuncture point and treat it with electrical microcurrents. Some patients report good results with this method of acupuncture.

If you try acupuncture, do so with your doctor's approval and make certain you go to a licensed practitioner who uses only disposable needles. You will probably go through a series of at least eight to ten treatments before deciding whether this is effective for you. You may not feel any relief for your breathing disorder, or you may feel extremely long-lasting relief. Acupuncture has very few contraindications, and the side effects are small if any. Certain disorders such as easy bleeding and local infection may preclude you from receiving acupuncture treatments.

Biofeedback

Biofeedback is a relaxation technique that uses electronics to measure such body responses associated with stress as heart rate or muscle contractions. This type therapy is based on the idea that when you are given information about your body's internal processes, you can use this information to learn to control those processes. It requires you to be connected to a machine that informs you and your therapist when you are physically relaxing your body. With sensors placed over specific muscle sites, the therapist will read the tension in your muscles, your heart rate, breathing pattern, amount of sweat produced, or body temperature. Any one or all of these readings can tell the trained biofeedback therapist whether you are learning to relax.

The ultimate goal of biofeedback is to use this skill outside the therapist's office when you are facing real stressors. If learned successfully, electronic biofeedback can help you control your heart rate, blood pressure, breathing patterns, and muscle tension when you are *not* hooked up to the machine. Some therapists recommend relaxation tapes that can be listened to at home to practice the relaxation techniques.

Although some recent studies on biofeedback for respiratory resistance, tracheal sounds, and vagal tone show hope, this complementary form of treatment needs further testing to prove its benefit in a management program. Thus, the clinical usefulness of biofeedback in dealing with breathing problems remains open to interpretation by your physician.

Hypnosis

Hypnosis is another alternative tool used to control stress. Although hypnosis comes from the Greek word meaning "sleep," it is really an intense state of focused concentration. This is not a new method of treatment, but it is now being used in innovative ways to improve the quality of life of respiratory patients.

In one controlled trial of chronic asthmatic patients who were inadequately controlled by drugs, after one year of hypnotherapy, the duration of hospitalization stays was reduced as well as the side effects of medications. More than 62 percent of the patients receiving hypnotherapy reported improvement in their symptoms, but measurements of air flow gave variable results.

If done correctly, this type of mind-body therapy can ideally produce a feeling of calm and improve a patient's confidence in handling the symptoms of a chronic breathing disorder. Because hypnosis is not meant for everyone, you should seek a qualified clinical psychologist or psychiatrist to help you decide whether hypnosis would be helpful and safe for you.

Homeopathic Medicine

Homeopathy is a therapeutic system of medicine that started in the late eighteenth century. It is based on the principle of "like cures like symptom." This means that remedies that would cause a potential problem in large doses would encourage the body to heal more rapidly if given in small doses.

Homeopathic remedies are highly diluted formulas of plant, mineral, and animal substances that can produce symptoms of the ailment in healthy people but alleviate similar symptoms in a sick person. The goal is to stimulate the body's reaction to throw off the offender.

Although homeopathic remedy sales are growing by 25 percent a year, according to the National Center for Homeopathy, this type of alternative medical treatment has always received great scrutiny by the traditional medical community. If you seek advice from a homeopathic practitioner, be sure this person is a medical doctor. Because of the possibility of allergic reactions, it is also imperative that you check with your own physician before taking any unknown substance or supplement that promises great cures.

Healing Foods and Herbs

If you have ever downed a cup of hot coffee and realized that it allowed you to breathe better, you have tried herbal medicine. According to the World Health Organization,

80 percent of the Earth's population uses plants to receive a desired benefit on the body.

However, there are some red flags that must be raised when attempting to improve breathing problems naturally. Although some herbs can have medicinal benefits, over-the-counter herbal preparations are not regulated by the U.S. government for safety. In other words, the word *natural* does not necessarily mean "safe." Some very popular herbal supplements have caused health problems, even death, in years past. Problems can arise from contamination during processing or even from the natural chemistry of the plant.

Some herbal preparations can affect your response to prescribed medication or may be toxic to your liver. Whatever new food or herbal preparation you choose to take, it is imperative to speak with your doctor or nutritionist before doing so to make sure that the product is safe and that no allergic reaction will result.

Caffeine

If you suffer from breathing problems, you probably know of the bronchodilator effects of caffeine. Although this is not a recommended means of treatment, one Canadian study reported in the *New England Journal of Medicine* found the bronchodilator effects of caffeine to be essentially the same as those of theophylline. These researchers suggested that in emergencies, several cups of strong coffee can help to relax contractions of the bronchioles in the lungs. A 120-pound person would have to ingest 2 cups of strong coffee to receive any bronchodilator effect (a 5-ounce cup of coffee contains 60 to 125 milligrams caffeine). Some allergic rhinitis sufferers also experience this relief. Preliminary studies report a strong cup of coffee eases stuffy noses and watery eyes.

On the other hand, be cautious of downing coffee if you are already on medication. Coffee may also intensify the side effects of theophylline or decongestants and cause a temporary increase in blood pressure, heart rate, anxiety, nervousness, or insomnia.

Foods High in Caffeine		
Coffee, drip	5 oz	90–115mg
Coffee, perk	5 oz	60–125mg
Coffee, instant	5 oz	60–80 mg
Coffee, decaf	5 oz	2–5 mg
Tea, 5-min steep	5 oz	40–100 mg
Tea, 3-min steep	5 oz	20–50 mg
Hot cocoa	5 oz	2–10 mg
Cola soft drink	12 oz	45 mg
Chocolate bar	1 oz	30 mg

Chicken Soup

Hot chicken soup, known also as Jewish penicillin, has been regarded for centuries as a "cure" for the common cold. Although research affirms that this is not a cure, hot chicken soup is a potent mucus stimulant, especially when it is loaded with pepper, garlic, hot curry powder, or other pungent spice that helps to thin out mucus in the mouth, throat, and lungs. (A discussion of mucus and cilia can be found on pages 7–8.)

Chicken also contains a natural amino acid called *cysteine,* which is similar in chemical content to a drug called acetylcysteine that doctors give for bronchitis and respiratory infections to help thin mucus and make it easier to eliminate.

Chili Peppers

Chili peppers are a great source of *capsaicin,* an antioxidant that also acts as a natural decongestant and expectorant. You can try chili peppers to season your foods or use a few drops of hot sauce in a food or beverage to open your sinuses and improve breathing.

Echinacea

Many studies from Germany suggest that this herb may mildly stimulate the immune system and help to ward off colds. Echinacea serves as a wound healer and anti-inflammatory, antiviral, and antibacterial herb. It is suggested that this herb be taken intermittently as its effectiveness wears off after eight weeks of continuous use. Although few side effects have been reported, asking your physician before trying it is vital. Echinacea may trigger allergic reactions in some people.

Garlic

Garlic, affectionately known as the stinking rose, has been called the most promising anticancer agent we have to date. The same elements that give garlic its powerful scent also give it its disease-preventing power.

Garlic appears to have antimicrobial and immunostimulating properties and may give some relief of symptoms of colds or upper respiratory problems. This occurs as garlic stimulates the mucus-producing vagus nerve reflexes.

You can find garlic in a variety of forms, including fresh, powder, and pills; however, raw garlic may be the most potent.

Ginger

Ginger has been used for medicinal purposes in China for thousands of years and may also act by stimulating mucus-producing vagus nerve reflexes. Ginger appears to have an antioxidant effect, as well as an anti-inflammatory effect, and stimulates the production of interferon which helps fight serious viral infections.

Goldenseal

This perennial herb is known for its action in soothing inflammation of the respiratory, digestive, and genitourinary tracts caused by allergy or infection. It also enhances mucous membrane function. Pregnant women, people with hypoglycemia, children, and the elderly are advised not to take this herb. Also, those who have pollen allergies should avoid this and similar herbs. Like echinacea, only take goldenseal for short periods.

Omega-3

Recent studies suggest that fish, fruit, and certain antioxidants help to give protection to the lungs. Researchers believe that eating high-fat fish, such as mackerel, cod, or salmon, that contain N-3 or omega-3 fatty acids enables the body to make more products that tend to decrease inflammation. Besides omega-3's, salmon is filled with calcium, magnesium, some carotenoids, complete proteins, and B vitamins. Vitamin B6 helps to boost the immune system and has been shown in preliminary studies to reduce some breathing problems.

Some patients with respiratory problems have found improvement in their breathing when they take these capsules for a few months. One revealing study in Australia found that the diets of children with asthma who ate fresh, oily fish such as tuna, herring, or salmon more than once a week had half the rate of asthma when compared with children who didn't. The researcher also reported that canned fish or fish cooked in oils did not have the same effect. Another study of dietary habits from researchers in the Netherlands revealed that the higher the consumption of fish along with such fruits as pears and apples, the lower the incidence of death from chronic obstructive pulmonary disease.

The most commonly available of these omega-3 fatty acids is found in some fish and fish oil. Although guidelines have not been established regarding supplements of fish oil, eicosapentaenoic acid (EPA) is available in capsules without a prescription. You can ask for these capsules at your drug or health food store. Check the instructions on the package label for the suggested dosage, and check with your doctor to see whether taking them would be detrimental to your condition. It is important to use EPA in addition to your prescribed medications, not to replace them. When used in the dose given on the label, no serious side effects are known at this time.

Vegetarians who want to gain this benefit can substitute borage seed oil, flaxseed oil, black currant seed oil, or evening primrose oil—all said to be helpful in offsetting inflammation. These oils all contain gammalinolenic acid (GLA), an omega-6 oil. One serving would be 2 tablespoons of flaxseed oil. This oil also has phytoestrogens, which have been linked to breast- and colon-cancer prevention.

High-Omega-3 Fish	
Anchovies	Salmon
Bluefish	Sardines
Capeline	Shad
Dogfish	Sturgeon
Herring	Tuna
Mackerel	Whitefish

Onions

Raw onions or scallions contain *quercetin*, a plant chemical that has been found to block allergic reactions by inhibiting the release of histamine and prostaglandins. Some researchers have found that eating onions or drinking onion juice may help reduce allergy-triggered asthma attacks or lessen bronchial asthma attacks. Onions, scallions, horseradish, radishes, and hot peppers all stimulate respiratory mucus production.

Thyme

Thyme contains *thymol*, which is a natural phytochemical. This immune-boosting herb has been used in antiseptic mouthwashes and herbal cough remedies. It is also used in herbal teas, especially for treating mild symptoms associated with coughs, cold, or flu.

Be Discerning and Safe

No matter how severe your symptoms are, perhaps the most important factor in gaining success with mind-body interplay is a belief that the treatment will work. This approach to wellness demands your personal involvement and commitment to improved health as you learn and do the various modes of therapy along with continuing the prescribed medications. Most importantly, using the mind-body modes of treatment forces you to be in touch with your body and your emotions and to listen to them. In many cases, simply understanding your body, your illness, and its accompanying symptoms will help you ward off a serious problem as you take action before a crisis occurs.

A word of caution must be stated. As you consider the different types of alternative treatments, it is of utmost importance to cautiously balance your desire to breathe easier with the dangers of the treatment, which may be unknown. Refrain from trying any remedies that promise quick relief but might be harmful. If you try a nonstandard or unproven treatment and there is no improvement, then you should stop that treatment. Often press reports make "breakthrough" treatments seem much more effective than they really are.

The most reasonable approach to any type of treatment—medical or complementary—is to know the *effects* and *side effects*. If you are suffering from shortness of breath or an infection that could be life threatening if ignored, traditional Western medicine manages this most effectively with medications. It is also excellent at providing an accurate diagnosis of your specific problem and treating breathing episodes or crises. Alternative treatment is beneficial when used to complement your physician's prescribed management plan as you learn to defuse your stress response, stay in a relaxed state of mind, and help boost your body's own healing power.

Check with your doctor before adding any type of alternative treatment to your breathing regime. Ask about the facts and seek honest, accurate information. Weigh the benefits and risks of any new remedy, just as you do when your doctor starts you on a new pill or inhaler. By being discerning, you can protect yourself from danger and be ready to benefit as early as possible from new discoveries.

Scientific Studies to Watch for in the Future

The National Institutes of Health (NIH) has recently opened an Office of Alternative Medicine (OAM). The OAM is funding current research at various institutions to *scientifically* evaluate the efficacy and safety of various alternative therapies.

Part 4

Special Situations

chapter 12

Ages and Stages

Pregnancy

If you are pregnant, you will experience many bodily changes that affect the functioning of your respiratory system. These include mechanical and biochemical factors. If you also have a respiratory disease, you may notice more change than usual in breathing and be faced with an increased risk of complications in the pregnancy as well as potentially adverse effects of your medicines on your fetus.

Breathlessness during Pregnancy

By the twelfth week of pregnancy, more than 20 percent of women have shortness of breath at rest and nearly 67 percent have this symptom on exertion. By the thirty-first week of gestation, 75 percent of expectant mothers have some breathlessness. This symptom may stem from the tendency to hyperventilate, or breathe faster than normal, because of the increased amounts of the hormone progesterone in circulation. Interestingly, unlike in obesity, the movement of the diaphragm is not impaired.

The Nose of the Expectant Mother

About one-half of all pregnant women have symptoms of rhinitis, both allergic and nonallergic, during gestation (see pages 18–20). This is caused by the increased blood volume during pregnancy, progesterone's effects on relaxing nasal blood vessels, and estrogen's effects on increasing the swelling of the lining membrane inside the nose. Nasal congestion will be worst during the second and third trimesters. Nasal polyps, sinusitis, and infectious rhinitis may be worsened due to the factors mentioned. Sinusitis occurs in about 1.5 percent of pregnant women. These problems can be severe enough to disturb sleep.

The treatment of nasal symptoms requires precise diagnosis, proper medicines, and in certain women, avoidance measures. (See the sections on treatment of nasal problems throughout this book for more information. For specific guidelines, note the tables on page 263.) Overall, an intranasal steroid such as beclomethasone, along with antihistamines, cromolyn, and antibiotics may be suggested and very helpful in your situation.

Smoking during Pregnancy

Studies of children have shown an association between passive exposure to maternal smoking and an increased frequency of acute respiratory illness and problems such as wheezing and asthma. One study compared healthy infants born to women who smoked in pregnancy with those born to women who did not smoke. Maternal smoking was associated with significant reductions in forced expiratory flow rates in the babies of women who smoked in pregnancy.

Of course, there must be no smoking, consumption of alcohol, and illicit drug usage during pregnancy.

Asthma in Pregnancy

The *Report of the Working Group on Asthma and Pregnancy* from the National Institutes of Health, 1993, recognizes that asthma is one of the most common diseases to complicate pregnancy. If you have asthma, be sure you have quality medical care to control lung function and to ensure that your baby receives an adequate supply of oxygen in the blood. When asthma is properly managed, the pregnancy and birth can go on with little or no increased risk to you or your baby. The goals of therapy for pregnant asthmatics are to prevent symptoms, maintain optimal pulmonary function, continue usual activity levels including exercise, avoid sudden episodes of worsening, avoid any adverse effects from asthma medications, and deliver a healthy infant.

Underestimation of asthma severity and undertreatment of exacerbations are two common errors that may lead to negative maternal or fetal results. Objective measures for assessing lung function are essential. The best is FEV-1, which is the volume of air that can be forcefully blown out in one second after taking a deep breath; it is convenient and reliable (page 69). Appropriate fetal monitoring is necessary, too.

Various reports note improvement of asthma during pregnancy in some women and worsening in others. A large study done in Finland indicated that asthma caused no emergencies during labor. There were no differences between asthmatic and nonasthmatic mothers with regard to the length of gestation, birth weight, incidences of prenatal deaths, neonatal respiratory problems, malformations, or low Apgar scores, a score that assesses the condition of a newborn according to heart rate, respiratory effort, color, muscle tone, and motor reactions. Severe asthma or systemic treatment (or both) during pregnancy did increase the incidence of preeclampsia (high blood pressure and possibly kidney problems) and low blood sugar levels in the mother. Among the asthmatic women, 28 percent had Caesarian sections compared with 17 percent in the nonasthmatic group of women.

Tuberculosis: Mother and Infant

Pregnancy neither predisposes to the development or progression of tuberculosis nor changes the usual symptoms and signs of the disease (pages 282–85). However, a recent increase in the rate of tuberculosis in the United States indicates that pregnant women have a higher chance of developing the disease.

You need to minimize any radiation hazards during your pregnancy. If your doctor suspects that you have tuberculosis, a chest X ray should be obtained after the twelfth week of gestation with your abdomen shielded. Radiographs should be done only if your tuberculosis skin test is positive and active tuberculosis needs to be ruled out. Skin testing is not a problem as it does not affect you or your baby. Antituberculosis therapy should be discussed with your doctor.

Obstructive Sleep Apnea

The prevalence of sleep apnea in pregnancy is unknown as are the effects of pregnancy on the severity of preexisting sleep apnea. However, sleep apnea may cause problems in the fetus because of the periods of low oxygen supply in the bloodstream. Early recognition and treatment of sleep apnea in pregnancy may avoid problems in the development of the fetus.

Cystic Fibrosis

With improved medical care, more and more people with cystic fibrosis (CF) will reach adulthood and want to start their own families. In a study of eleven pregnancies in eight women with CF, the mother's health worsened during and after pregnancy and did not return to baseline after delivery. If you have CF and are thinking of starting a family, be sure you have excellent nutritional and pulmonary evaluations which will help in determining any risks.

Preferred Drugs for Respiratory Problems during Pregnancy or Breastfeeding

DRUG CLASS	DRUG NAME
Anti-inflammatory	Cromolyn sodium
	Beclomethasone
	Prednisone
Bronchodilator	Inhaled beta2-agonist
	Theophylline
Antihistamine	Chlorpheniramine
	Tripelennamine
Decongestant	Pseudoephedrine
	Oxymetazoline
Cough	Guaifenesin
	Dextromethorphan
Antibiotics	Amoxicillin (if *not* allergic to penicillin)
	Erythromycin
	Isoniazid
	Rifampin
	Ethambutol

Medications to Avoid during Pregnancy and Breastfeeding

Alpha-adrenergic compounds (other than pseudoephedrine)	Pyrazinamide
	Streptomycin
Epinephrine	Aminoglycosides
Iodides	Coumadin
Sulfonamines (in late pregnancy)	Flu vaccine
Tetracyclines	Pneumovax
Quinalones	

Other Lung Infections

During pregnancy, you may be more susceptible to pneumonia caused by the virus that causes chickenpox. This is called varicella pneumonia and can be particularly severe during pregnancy.

A fungal infection that causes a certain type of pneumonia and can be contracted in the southwestern United States is called coccidiomycosis. It can be very severe in pregnant women, especially if caught during the pregnancy.

Young Children

Because all children deserve to be healthy enough for exercise, activity, and regular school attendance, getting an accurate diagnosis of any respiratory disease is important. The goals of treatment for a young child with a respiratory system disorder include maintaining normal lung function so that the child may participate in a lifestyle that is conducive to normal growth and development.

The Struggle to Breathe

Infants and young children have many respiratory problems. Perhaps one of the most serious problems occurs in some premature infants. Although the bronchi are formed by the sixteenth week of gestation, the air sacs are not ready to exchange gas until at least the twenty-eighth week of gestation. Infants born prematurely often struggle to breathe because their air sacs are not fully developed. These infants are said to have *respiratory distress syndrome* and frequently require high concentrations of oxygen to survive.

Prompt recognition of the problem and use of the respirator and oxygen will save the premature infant's life. These treatments can sometimes cause an injury to the lungs called *bronchopulmonary dysplasia (BPD)*. Some infants with BPD require supplemental oxygen at home until their lungs have healed sufficiently. Except in rare cases, BPD is not associated with permanent lung disease, and most of these children have normal lung function when they get older. Over the past two decades, advances in medical treatment of respiratory distress syndrome have reduced the severity of BPD and greatly improved the quality of life of these infants.

Apnea

Apnea (cessation of breathing), or Sudden Infant Death Syndrome (SIDS), is another serious complication of prematurity. Under normal circumstances breathing is controlled by the respiratory centers in the brain. But these centers need a full-term pregnancy to mature properly.

Premature infants can have apnea, which is a prolonged interruption in the regular respiratory rate. Some babies may benefit from a special monitor at home to alert a parent that there is a problem. Apnea can also occur in children with certain infections, but this is not as common.

Birth Defects

Birth defects or congenital malformations occur when there has been a problem in the early formation of a structure in the respiratory system. Minor anatomical defects in the nose, throat, or breathing tubes generally do not cause any noticeable problems. However, severe narrowing of the bronchial tubes, particularly the larger tubes, can result in significant respiratory distress needing immediate attention. Sometimes surgery is necessary to correct the problem.

Respiratory Infections

Healthy term babies have the same respiratory patterns as adults although babies typically have a faster rate of breathing. Respiratory infections such as pneumonia are common in babies and are usually associated with coughing and fever. Other infections cause inflammation of the small breathing tubes. This condition is called *bronchiolitis*. The main symptom of bronchiolitis is wheezing, which usually ends in a few days. Some infants may become seriously ill and require hospitalization. Most cases of bronchiolitis occur during the winter in the first year of life and are caused by viruses.

Antibiotics are not used in the treatment of bronchiolitis although bronchodilators to relieve wheezing may be helpful. One case of bronchiolitis does not necessarily protect an infant from getting a repeat infection. It has been observed that bronchiolitis in infants is associated with a higher incidence of asthma in older children. This has researchers questioning whether exposure to certain viruses in early life predisposes children to asthma later.

Croup

Between the ages of six and thirty-six months, children are susceptible to croup. This illness is also caused by a viral infection, usually parainfluenza, which causes inflammation and swelling of the windpipe or trachea in the area below the vocal cords. Children with croup have a characteristic cough that sounds like the bark of a seal. Croup usually requires no treatment and lasts for a few days, although some children have such difficulty breathing that they are treated in the hospital. Such children may be given racemic epinephrine by aerosolized mist and a short course of intravenous steroids to relieve the swelling.

Strep Throat

A sore throat with or without fever may suggest an infection due to Streptococcus or a virus. A definitive diagnosis should be made using a special Q-tip for swabbing the throat to culture the specific bacteria responsible for the problem. Strep throat is easily treatable with appropriate antibiotics such as penicillin or erythromycin for penicillin-allergic patients. Severe and recurrent strep throat may be an indication for tonsillectomy.

Bacterial Pneumonia

Bacterial pneumonia refers to an infection of the lung and is usually associated with fever, chills, cough, and chest pain. The diagnosis is confirmed by a chest X ray. The most common cause is a bacteria called Streptococcus pneumoniae, which is easily treated by antibiotics. *Walking pneumonia* refers to an infection by Mycoplasma pneumoniae, and infected children are usually mildly ill with a low-grade fever and cough. A chest X ray and blood test confirm the diagnosis. Children are given specific antibiotics for these infections.

Asthma

It is estimated that as many as 10 percent of all children have asthma at some time during their childhood. This lung disease can affect infants as well as older children. As the most common chronic childhood disease, asthma causes more hospital admissions and visits to the emergency room than any other illness, and the prevalence of asthma is increasing. In the United States, the increase in asthma prevalence has predominantly affected children younger than seventeen years. Although environmental factors such as air pollution and increased exposure to aeroallergens have been implicated, precise reasons for this trend remain unclear.

Asthma is characterized by inflammation of the bronchial tubes, production of sticky secretions inside the breathing tubes, and contraction of the muscle that spirals around the bronchial tubes. Not all children with asthma wheeze. Chronic cough may be the only obvious sign, and a child's asthma may go unrecognized if the cough is attributed to recurrent bronchitis. Pulmonary function tests cannot be done on very young children.

Typically, your child's asthma will flare because of triggers. The most common triggers are viral respiratory infections, cold air, exercise, exposure to environmental tobacco smoke, and allergies. Not all children with allergies have asthma, but an allergy to house dust mites and cockroaches can be particularly problematic. Measures to reduce the infestation of mites and cockroaches in the environment, as described in Chapter 6, are frequently helpful in reducing asthma symptoms. When possible, avoiding allergens is a simple way to help control allergy and asthma symptoms. Immunotherapy (allergy shots), as discussed on pages 116–17, may be used in some children, although there are new questions about whether allergy shots benefit a child's asthma.

Environmental tobacco smoke is an important trigger, and parents should make certain that their child is not exposed to it. Smoking around the child should not be permitted, especially in confined places such as the child's bedroom or a car.

Successful treatment of asthma is based on the selection of appropriate medicines which are quite similar to those used in adults (see Chapter 5). Some medications are designed to provide *relief* from asthma symptoms, whereas others are used to *prevent* asthma symptoms from developing. Your child needs a treatment program tailored to her or his individual needs. This includes extensive education of both parent and child. You should learn how and when to assess your child for early signs of asthma symptoms. Emergency room treatment can often be avoided if you can recognize these signs and intervene early with appropriate medications. Although childhood asthma generally improves over time, about 10 percent of children have severe asthma requiring chronic use of medication including steroids.

Cystic Fibrosis

Cystic fibrosis (CF) is an inherited disease characterized by chronic cough and infections of the lung. It occurs more commonly in Caucasians than other races. In order to develop CF, your child must receive the CF gene from both parents. For example, if your infant has two CF genes on chromosome number seven, she would be diagnosed with CF. It is *very important* to recognize that inadequate or inappropriate prenatal care does *not* play a role in whether a child has CF.

The common symptoms of cystic fibrosis include a persistent cough, recurrent pneumonia, stunted growth, nasal obstruction or drip, and sinusitis. Nasal polyps may occur in as many as 20 percent of children with CF. The bronchial mucus becomes very thick, tenacious, and greenish if infected with various bacteria. Sometimes a bacteria called pseudomonas grows in the mucus. About one-half of those with CF have a fungus called aspergillus in their sputum. Some may have a species of bacteria related to tuberculosis.

In young children, the smaller bronchial tubes are obstructed early on in CF. Your doctor can detect this problem in your child by using spirometry, as discussed in Chapter 4. As the disease progresses, your child may have asthma or COPD-like symptoms.

If your doctor suspects that your child has CF, he or she will perform a sweat test in which sweat is analyzed chemically. Children with a high concentration of chloride in their sweat and significant symptoms are likely to have CF. Certain DNA evaluations or genetic analysis may be helpful, too.

Since the basic problem of CF involves the mucosal lining layers of the bronchial tubes, as well as other tubes or ducts in sweat glands, gallbladder, and pancreas, there may be coincidental symptoms related to these organs. The pancreas may not be able to secrete certain digestive juices that it normally does. The gallbladder may become inflamed and even develop gallstones. The chronic bacterial bronchitis causes an intense destructive inflammatory response that results in damage to the airway.

Therapies for Cystic Fibrosis

Newer forms of therapy offer great hope to those with CF. Some treatments involve special agents to thin and mobilize the thick mucus seen in CF. Perhaps the most effective treatment uses an enzyme that helps disintegrate the remains of the inflammatory cells in the mucus. It is called DNAase and has been shown to decrease episodes of worsening that require hospitalization. DNAase reduces the need to use powerful antibiotics for complications with infections, and it can also provide sustained improvement in pulmonary function.

DNAase is delivered to the airways by inhalation, and the only consistent adverse reactions have been laryngitis and hoarseness. Your child may benefit from this therapy, although the cost is still very high.

Because CF is caused by a genetic mutation, research directed at dealing with this is ongoing and shows great promise. For those who develop respiratory failure, a lung transplant is a consideration. If both lungs are transplanted, the survival rate is high. Breakthrough methods in understanding this disease may bring genetic engineering or medicines to control the underlying defect in this disease in the near future.

Emotional Concerns

Having a chronic respiratory problem is difficult for anyone. Nevertheless, when your child has difficulty breathing, this causes added emotional stress for the entire family. Especially if your child's breathing problem is not well managed, it is not unusual to revolve your entire life around the chronically ill child. In doing so, you may ignore your own needs as well as the needs of others in the family.

As you may have experienced, taking time away from your role as parent-nurse may be infrequent. Many parents express normal fears that the child may suffer a breathing problem or react to a new allergen in a strange environment if they are not around. Living day after day with unending anxiety stemming from the real fear that the child will not breathe normally can frequently lead to feelings of sadness or even hopelessness. As one mother said, "I can never be off duty. It is as if I am on red alert twenty-four hours a day, every day, in case my child has a problem."

How does a respiratory problem affect the child? He can become equally dependent on the parent, usually the mother. Such normal childhood activities as attending birthday parties, joining sports teams, or even playing out-of-doors with peers may be limited for fear the child will have breathing problems or catch someone's cold. The child may be restricted to playing indoors for fear of having an allergic reaction to pollen, plants, or grass or for fear of weather changes that effect breathing. The family may hesitate to take vacations as an emergency could arise and the child's doctor might be needed. This further ties the child to the parent and hinders independent development.

If your child has respiratory problems, even more anxiety is experienced when she leaves for the first day of school. You wonder if this will be the day her asthma worsens. Thoughts run through your mind, such as "What if she has an emergency, and I am not at home? Will her teacher know what to do? How will she breathe if she cannot find her inhaler? What if they serve cookies made of wheat or eggs? What if there is a gerbil in the classroom? What if the school nurse cannot find her Epipen (epinephrine)?" Living year after year with these fears and anxieties is bound to create a weakened emotional state for you and your child.

When a chronically ill child does start school, another problem arises with absenteeism, making up class work, and staying up with grade-level skills. For instance, asthma is one of the leading causes of sickness-related absenteeism from school.

Taking Control

Knowing that a chronic respiratory problem is bound to change your life and the life of your child, it is important to realize that control is crucial. This control varies from person to person, depending on the severity of the illness. However, the ultimate goal is for you and your child to live a normal life without experiencing major symptoms.

Learn all you can about your child's particular problem, and let her doctor instruct you in prevention measures, such as how to use a peak flow meter (pages 70–1) and how to use a spacer (pages 101–2). As your child matures, teach her about her illness and encourage personal responsibility in using medications and understanding symptoms. Talk openly with her close friends, and tell them what the warning signs are. Ask them to remind her to take any preventive or treatment medications if she is away from home. If she has food allergies, make sure she understands the importance of allergic food avoidance, as well as the avoidance of other personal allergens such as animals, dust, or mold.

Openly communicate about your child's problem with family members, grandparents, neighbors, teachers, babysitters, bus drivers, or anyone who will be responsible for your child when he is out of your care. Give caretakers material about the problem, including the list of warning signs, and teach them how to use the appropriate treatment, whether nebulizer, inhaler, or medication. Some parents find it helpful to give their child's caretaker a pager. The pager allows the caretaker to dial an access code and reach the parent within minutes should an emergency arise or there be a concern.

Stay in touch with other parents who are faced with the same problems. A parent support group can offer comfort and empathy, and parents usually have a wealth of prevention and treatment ideas. Check with your pediatrician to see whether a support group meets in your area, or join with several parents you know and form your own.

Prevention and Detection

Once you are aware of risk factors and symptoms for specific problems common in young children, you can take proactive steps to eliminate those over which you have control, while seeking medical attention. With early prevention and detection of respiratory disorders, when treatment is most effective, young children can have the hope of maintaining proper lung development and living full, active lives.

Older Adults

No one escapes the changes that come with age. Sometimes it is difficult for a physician to distinguish aging from disease, as they commonly coexist.

Even in normal healthy adults, the lungs show some specific changes with maturity. Changes that occur in the small air sacs and airways throughout the lungs make them less efficient. The level of oxygen in the blood slowly decreases with age in a predictable way. The changes happen in people who have no lung problems and who do not smoke.

Yet, changes associated with aging should *not* include shortness of breath at rest or with activity. When these symptoms occur, a medical evaluation is indicated and treatment is warranted.

Natural Decline in Function

Aging is associated with progressive structural and physiological changes that produce a decline in function. Diseases that affect the respiratory tract will further speed this decline, as well as environmental factors such as smoking, pollutants, and lack of regular exercise. Problems in other organ systems, such as the heart, can also make it more difficult to breathe normally.

With age-related pulmonary functional decline, you may find it more difficult to get over an infection. Years of cigarette smoking or contact with toxic chemicals can lead to serious illnesses such as emphysema, bronchitis, lung cancer, or certain kinds of inflammation in the lungs (interstitial diseases). These diseases can further compromise the lung function.

Many new prevention and treatment measures can work to manage lung disease. That is why it is important to recognize any symptoms or bodily changes when they first occur so you can start effective treatment in the earliest stages when it can do the most good.

Anatomical and Functional Changes

Interestingly, functional impairment from disease is easier to treat with drugs than are impairments due to aging. However, older adults need to use caution taking any type of drug because their liver and kidneys cannot process drugs as quickly as younger adults. This creates a greater threat of adverse reactions and drug overdoses in older adults.

For example, asthma is reversible with appropriate medications. In contrast, anatomical emphysema is due to *age-related* loss of normally elastic lung tissue. Breathing at rest is totally dependent on the elastic recoil of the inflated lung and the cross-sectional diameter of the airways. The age-related decline in respiratory function is partly due to the loss of elastic recoil, as well as diaphragmatic, chest wall, and abdominal wall weakness. A discussion of lung structure, elastic recoil, and emphysema may be found on page 42.

As we age, there is a generalized change in the elastic tissue of the lung, which causes *panlobular emphysema*. Panlobular emphysema is commonly known as emphysema of the nonsmoker elderly. Fortunately, these changes may not significantly impair breathing.

In contrast, an older adult who is a chronic smoker develops *centrilobular emphysema*. This type of emphysema is an inflammatory disorder of the airway tubes (bronchioles) that leads to the distention and rupture of the lungs (alveolus) and could adversely affect breathing. Both types of emphysema can affect a person who smokes.

Inflammation and aging of the lungs lead to a decline in the ability to get oxygen from the atmosphere into the bloodstream. This can be further compromised in the presence of a weak heart; an older adult who has a lung disorder and develops a heart attack commonly ends up in the intensive care unit with serious respiratory problems.

The chest wall is another important anatomic component for breathing. The bony thorax, diaphragm, and abdominal muscles are the major components of the chest wall. During relaxed breathing only the diaphragm is actively contributing to the breathing process. During exertion other muscles contribute for a higher volume of air exchange.

With advancing age, respiratory muscles decrease in size and condition. The decrease results in a reduction of aerobic capacity and endurance. The older adult may feel such symptoms as shortness of breath and easy fatiguability during exertion. Those who are overweight also have a restriction of air exchange because of the increased work the diaphragm must do against a large, heavy abdomen. In addition, older adults with deconditioned respiratory muscles have difficulty withstanding the increased demands of breathing associated with infections such as bronchitis or pneumonia.

As discussed in Chapter 7, with training and regular aerobic exercises, respiratory muscles can be strengthened and endurance improved so that breathing capacity is maintained and improved. Older adults who are sedentary, especially those who are bed or chair bound, are very prone to developing serious respiratory illness, and, after recovery from a respiratory illness, commonly show a significant decline in their ability to take care of themselves. In contrast, those seniors who remain physically active and exercise regularly tend to survive a respiratory problem with *less* decline in function.

Common Respiratory Diseases

Asthma in older adults has the same symptoms as previously discussed on pages 45–57. However, with increasing age, the choice of medications will differ as there is a decrease in the beta2-receptor function. These receptors are important for maintaining the caliber of the bronchial tubes.

Such beta2-stimulant inhalers as albuterol (Ventolin), commonly prescribed for younger asthmatics, may not be effective in the elderly. Those who are sensitive to acetylcholine may benefit from the use of anticholinergic drugs such as ipratropium (Atrovent). Although many doctors still prescribe inhaled beta2-agonists for asthma, it is common to combine both the beta2-agonist and the anticholinergic inhaler in a comprehensive treatment plan.

Chronic obstructive pulmonary disease (COPD) and asthma may be difficult to distinguish in older adults. Chronic bronchitis and emphysema generally coexist and are frequently associated with chronic smoking or environmental exposure. With COPD, the cellular changes in the lining of the airways are obvious, and the reversibility depends on the degree of change. Your response to medications can be monitored using spirometry. You should also note how frequently you cough and your mucus volume.

Pneumonia in older adults is commonly caused by a bacteria called Streptococcus pneumoniae that usually responds to an antibiotic such as penicillin or erythromycin. As discussed, the pneumococcal vaccine can potentially prepare your body to fight this bacteria. For those who live in a nursing home, retirement home, or hospital, there are often different and more aggressive bacteria that usually require more expensive antibiotics. Your doctor can guide you toward the best treatment.

Influenza is a respiratory illness common to all ages. However, this virus tends to affect older adults more detrimentally. Influenza type A is more virulent than type B. Both can lead to pneumonia in older adults, and pneumonia is the fourth leading cause of death in the United States for those over age seventy. Although an annual influenza vaccine is highly recommended, the antibody response in an older person to the influenza vaccine is considerably less than 80 percent of the protection in a healthy young person.

If you are an older adult, do not take the vaccine, and are exposed to the flu, a medication called *amantadine* can be used. If you take this drug within forty-eight hours of the onset of symptoms, amantadine reduces the duration of symptoms of influenza nearly 50 percent. You may have difficulty tolerating amantadine and experience such feelings as lightheadedness or weakness. Stay in contact with your doctor while you take this.

Tuberculosis may be reactivated and is commonly observed in nursing home patients who had exposure to the disease in the past. In fact, a startling 80 percent of older adults in the United States are infected with tuberculosis. The reason for this high statistic is that seniors today were children when the bacteria that causes tuberculosis was common. Of those infected, many developed the disease in young adulthood. However, some did not and now develop a reactivation of the disease. Immunosenescence, or a decline in immune defenses with age, appears to reduce the ability of older people to resist this reactivation of tuberculosis. (See the discussion of tuberculosis on pages 282–85).

Pulmonary embolism commonly occurs in the less active or bed-bound elderly or after any major orthopedic surgery. It involves the development of blood clots in the veins of the lower extremities. These blood clots may break off and circulate back to the right side of the heart. From there, they may be pumped into the lungs where they block blood vessels, damage the lung, and produce problems with gas exchange. Pulmonary embolism can cause shortness of breath and decreased exercise tolerance.

Lung cancer can be affected by increasing age because of the longer duration of exposure to inhaled carcinogens such as cigarette smoke. A decline in immunity also increases the susceptibility to this disease.

As we have emphasized, with any respiratory symptom, get an early and accurate diagnosis so your doctor can differentiate between the normal decline of aging and an infection or serious disease. Once the diagnosis is made, there are many types of breakthrough medical treatments that can help you breathe comfortably, as well as allow you to stay active with a good quality of life.

chapter 13

Serious Diseases

AIDS

Over a half million cases of the Acquired Immuno-deficiency Syndrome (AIDS) were reported in the United States by November 1995. Though more than 300,000 have since died, hope for long-term survival increases daily. Newer drugs can fight the Human Immuno-deficiency Virus (HIV) which causes AIDS. Recent success in combining medical treatments gives great promise in keeping the immune system healthy. Although there is not yet a cure, new scientific discoveries are being made that give hope for this happening in the future.

Early in the AIDS epidemic, those at the highest risk were homosexual and bisexual men. More recently, intra-venous drug users who share needles and people with whom they have unprotected sexual activity have become the most likely victims of the disease.

If you are infected with HIV, you may experience a progressive deterioration of your immune function over a period of years. Respiratory diseases, particularly lung infections, are the major causes of illness and death.

The severity of weakening of your immune defenses

determines the development of respiratory disorders. The most useful measure of immune defense is the number of special white cells called *CD4 lymphocytes*. Although common problems like sinusitis and bronchitis may occur at any CD4 cell count, bacterial pneumonia and tuberculosis occur when this cell count is lower. Decreased immunity can lead to infection with a protozoa called pneumocystis carinii, a virus known as cytomegalovirus (CMV), atypical mycobacteria, fungal infections, and an unusual tumor, Kaposi's sarcoma.

Streptococcus pneumonia, Hemophilus influenza, and Pseudomonas are recognized as the most common causes of pneumonia in those infected with HIV. If you have this bacterial pneumonia, you may experience symptoms such as fever, chills, and cough productive of yellow, green, or bloody phlegm. There are specific antibiotics used to treat this problem. If you have a low CD4 cell count, the pneumonia vaccine, Pneumovax, is highly recommended.

After the protozoa called pneumocystis carinii harbors silently for a period of time, the symptoms of this infection come on suddenly. You may have increasing shortness of breath over weeks, even months. Sometimes the symptoms occur suddenly with quick worsening over a few days. You may or may not have fever, and you may also have an infection, called thrush, on the tongue due to Candida, a fungus.

The chest X ray is an important tool for determining whether this infection is present. Your doctor will confirm the diagnosis by examining your sputum or special washes from the lung.

Specific antibiotics and corticosteroids are important in bringing the infection and associated inflammation under control. Prophylactic use of the antibiotic combination trimethoprim-sulfamethoxazole (TMP-SMX) may prevent infection and help to prolong your life.

Mild reductions in the immune defenses associated with small decreases in CD4 cell counts increase the risk of reactivation of tuberculosis. This infection runs a more aggressive course in AIDS patients. Your doctor will diagnose this by looking for mycobacteria in your sputum or in specimens from your lung. Sometimes medications may be started on the basis of the chest-X-ray appearance while the sputum culture is pending.

As with all respiratory problems, it is important that you seek prompt treatment for tuberculosis. This will improve the success rate of stopping the infection and reduce the transmission of the disease to other people.

Various fungal infections may also cause you to experience severe lung problems. The most common is cryptococcus. Here, meningitis usually occurs simultaneously. Other fungal infections that may cause serious problems are Histoplasmosis, especially in those who live in areas near the Ohio and Mississippi river valleys, and Coccidiomycoses, in the southwestern United States.

If you have an advanced HIV infection, you may suffer with chronic bronchitis and bronchiectasis even if you never smoked. Certain kinds of inflammatory diseases of the lung may occur and may be confused with infectious diseases.

The good news is that our ability to treat infectious complications of AIDS has greatly improved. However, scientists are now faced with more difficult respiratory problems, some of which resist treatment. Until an effective vaccine, drug therapy, or cure is discovered, the best management of HIV infection remains avoidance by following safe sexual practices and hygienic lifestyles.

Tuberculosis

As discussed on pages 262 and 278, tuberculosis is now being seen more frequently, especially among older adults and AIDS patients. The discovery of effective antibiotics and the institution of measures to control the spread of tuberculosis (TB) resulted in a decreasing number of new cases until about 1985. At that time, the trend was reversed due to the increase in AIDS sufferers. Tuberculosis is also a frequent cause of death in North America among older adults, inner-city poor, and minority groups. In recent years, the infection has been seen even more in nursing homes.

Approximately 10 million Americans have been infected by the agent that causes TB, and an astounding *one-third of the world's population* is infected with TB. This infection probably accounts for about 6 percent of deaths worldwide.

Tuberculosis is an infection caused by a bacteria called Mycobacterium tuberculosis which likes to live and reproduce in people's lungs. The bacteria can multiply in areas of the lung where the most destruction takes place due to the body's attempts to contain the infection by an inflammatory response involving special blood cells. These areas of the lung may become filled with partially liquified debris containing the tuberculosis bacteria which can be coughed out into the surrounding air. If a healthy person inhales liquid droplets containing the infectious agent, the disease may be contracted. Since the droplets are generally few in number and may contain only few bacteria, it usually takes many months of close exposure as in a household or nursing home to spread the disease.

The degree of infectiousness depends on the number of bacteria in the expectorated sputum and the frequency of the cough. Good ventilation is an essential part of preventing the spread of the disease. Interestingly, mycobacteria are easily killed by ultraviolet light so transmission of the disease rarely occurs in daylight.

In the United States, 90 percent of normal people who

are infected do not develop tuberculous because their immune systems are able to contain and control the infectious agents. When tuberculosis bacteria enter the lung, they are ingested by defender cells called macrophages and taken to local lymph nodes which act as filters. Occasionally the mycobacteria are not held in these lymph nodes but get into the bloodstream and are transported throughout the body. The bacteria end up in areas such as the liver, kidney, bone, brain, or other parts of the lung. Although most of these areas heal, they may cause problems later in life if the infected person becomes weakened with age, malnutrition, or a compromised immune system, as in AIDS.

The initial infection usually does not cause symptoms, but if it spreads throughout the body initially or is reactivated later, it may cause fever, weight loss, and night sweats as well as a cough. The cough may be dry, hacking, or productive of blood-streaked phlegm. Sometimes the infection breaks through the lining of the lung and causes an inflammatory reaction in the space between the lung and the chest wall. This is called pleuritis and may be associated with sharp chest pain worsened by breathing movements. Destructive diseases due to inflammation may occur in many parts of the body.

Diagnosis

The diagnosis of tuberculosis depends on symptoms such as a cough or an abnormal chest X ray; certain chest-X-ray appearances are highly suggestive of TB. Skin testing may play an important role in making the diagnosis.

Treatment

The treatment of tuberculosis requires a combination of effective antimycobacterial drugs. You may need more than one drug to prevent the multiplication of drug-resistant bacteria. The most important drugs are isoniazid, rifampin, pyrazinamide, and ethambutol. Therapy must be done under the close supervision of an experienced physician. Sometimes, one drug alone, isoniazid, may be sufficient to prevent the development of the disease in certain individuals who have been infected. There is a vaccine for the prevention of tuberculosis which is recommended by the Centers for Disease Control and Prevention for certain children and health care workers who are at high risk of exposure to TB. This vaccine is called BCG and uses live, weakened mycobacteria to stimulate immune defenses in high-risk groups.

Interstitial Lung Disease

The earliest symptoms of interstitial lung diseases, which are peculiar inflammations of the lung, are shortness of breath during exercise and a dry cough with no obvious cause. Almost 200 known different diseases are associated with these kinds of lung inflammation that involve the walls of the alveoli and the surrounding lung structures. Some of the related diseases have a known cause while others do not. Common identifiable causes include occupational and environmental exposures due to various dusts and gases. Sometimes certain drugs or medicines themselves may be causative. Prompt diagnosis is important because the sooner therapy is started the more likely worsening of the disease will be slowed down or halted.

Symptoms mentioned above call for a physical examination, which may reveal characteristic noises in the lungs heard with a stethoscope and typical abnormalities shown by a chest X ray. Pulmonary function testing may show evidence of reduced lung volumes and other functional problems. A physician who takes a sufficiently detailed medical history from the patient with these findings may order specialized blood tests and a computerized chest X ray, or CT scan, to better define the situation; often a biopsy, or sampling of a piece of the lung itself, is needed to distinguish one cause from another.

Once the diagnosis is completed, treatment may be started. The most commonly used medicine is prednisone, which is valuable for its anti-inflammatory properties. A patient with interstitial lung disease should be under the care of an experienced pulmonologist.

Lung Cancer

Lung cancer is the leading cause of cancer deaths in the United States. It affects more than 100,000 men and 50,000 women each year. The majority of these people die within one year of diagnosis. Most lung cancer occurs between ages fifty-five and sixty-five. The overall incidence is increasing, even though antismoking campaigns begun more than twenty years ago have slowed the rate a bit in white males. Unfortunately, the rate in females is increasing. Even for those whose cancer is apparently confined to the lung without spread to other parts of the body, the chance of being alive after five years is only 30 percent for men and 50 percent for women.

The vast majority of lung cancers are caused by cigarette smoking. The overall relative risk of getting lung cancer increases ten to fifteen times by active smoking and about two times by long-term inhalation of second-hand smoke. The risk is magnified sixty to seventy times in a man who has smoked two packs each day for twenty years. The chance of getting lung cancer diminishes after quitting but *may never* return to the nonsmoker level. The rise in lung cancer among women is due to the increasing number of them who smoke.

The optimal treatment is prevention. Ideally, tobacco smoke should *never* be inhaled. Efforts to get people to stop smoking are of paramount urgency. Overcoming the powerful addiction to nicotine is a challenge that usually requires support of family, friends, and professionals as well as nicotine-containing smoke substitutes such as chewing gum, special medicine patches, and occasionally, temporary use of tranquilizers.

Symptoms of lung cancer that should bring a person to the attention of a doctor include an annoying cough, particularly if producing bloody mucus, a wheeze localized to one side of the chest, or a pneumonia that fails to respond appropriately to antibiotics. Chest X rays are extremely valuable in the diagnosis of lung cancer. The best chance for cure occurs when small tumors, localized in a lung, are found and can be cut out by a surgeon. When patients are not candidates for surgery because of one problem or another, radiation therapy or chemotherapy (with special medicines) may be helpful in individual cases.

Pulmonary Hypertension

Primary pulmonary hypertension is a rare disease associated with high blood pressures in the arteries that go from the right side of the heart to the lungs. There is no obvious cause. Symptoms that occur early on include trouble breathing during exercise in an otherwise healthy person. The disease is twice as common in women. Treatment is very difficult and rarely successful.

Secondary pulmonary hypertension is similar to primary but has some identifiable causes such as certain kinds of heart disease, various lung diseases, and the use of certain drugs. Aminorex fumarate (Menocil), a popular drug used in the 1960s through the 1980s by overweight people to help them lose weight, caused pulmonary hypertension in many of its users. In April 1996, the Food and Drug Administration approved dexfenfluramine (Redux) for use in the United States. Several large weight-loss franchises began marketing this prescription drug in combination with traditional diet and exercise programs. Subsequently, the *New England Journal of Medicine* published an article describing the findings of the International Pulmonary Hypertension Study Group, which showed a 23-fold increase in the risk of developing pulmonary hypertension for those who used Redux more than three months. (Menocil caused a tenfold increase.) Dexfenfluramine usage will lead to a sustained although small weight loss. The risk of using this drug must be weighed against the benefits. Some experts warn that if someone has a genetic predisposition, Redux may trigger the development of pulmonary hypertension. Recent onset of shortness of breath with strenuous activity, in spite of weight loss, is a warning sign.

Part 5

Resources

Support Organizations

Allergy and Asthma Network
Mothers of Asthmatics
3554 Chain Bridge Road, Suite 200
Fairfax, VA 22030
(703) 385–4403

Alpha-1 National Foundation
1829 Portland Avenue
Minneapolis, MN
(612) 871–1747

American Academy of Allergy, Asthma & Immunology
(AAAAI)
611 East Wells Street
Milwaukee, WI 53202
(414) 272–6071
(800) 822–ASMA (2762)

American Academy of Environmental Medicine
P.O. Box CN1001–8001
New Hope, PA 18938
(215) 862–4544

American Academy of Medical Acupuncture
5820 Wilshire Boulevard, Suite 500
Los Angeles, CA 90036
(800) 521–AAMA

American Academy of Pediatrics
141 Northwest Point Boulevard
P.O. Box 927
Elk Grove Village, IL 60009–0927
(847) 228–5005

American Association of Certified Allergists (AACA)
85 West Algonquin Road, Suite 550
Arlington Heights, IL 60005

American Association of Oriental Medicine
433 Front Street
Catasauqua, PA 18032
(610) 266–1433

American Association of Respiratory Care
11030 Ables Lane
Dallas, TX 75229–4593

American College of Allergy and Immunology
800 East Northwest Highway, Suite 1080
Palatine, IL 60067
(708) 359–2800
(800) 842–7777

American Dietetic Association
National Center for Nutrition and Dietetics
216 West Jackson Boulevard
Chicago, IL 60606–6995
Nutritional Hotline (800) 366–1655

American Lung Association
1740 Broadway
New York, NY 10019
(800) 586–4872

American Sleep Disorders Association
1610 14 Street, Northwest, Suite 300
Rochester, MN 55901

Asthma and Allergy Foundation of America (AAFA)
1125 15 Street, NW, Suite 502
Washington, DC 20005
(800) 624–0044
(800) 7–ASTHMA [(800) 727–8462]

Cystic Fibrosis Foundation
6931 Arlington Road
Bethesda, MD 20814
(800) 344–4823

Food Allergy Network
10400 Eaton Place, Suite 107
Fairfax, VA 22030–2208
(703) 691–3179

Manitoba Lung Association
629 McDermot Avenue
Winnipeg, Manitoba, CAN R3A 1P6
(204) 774–5501

National Association of Managed Care Professionals
(NAMCP)
4435 Waterfront Drive, Suite 101
Glen Allen, VA 23060
(800) 722–0376

National Asthma Education and Prevention Program of
the National Heart, Lung, and Blood Institute
P.O. Box 30105
Bethesda, MD 20824–0105
(301) 251–1222

National Commission for the Certification of
Acupuncturists
1424 16 Street, NW, Suite 501
Washington, DC 20036
(202) 232–1404

National Jewish Center for Immunology and Respiratory
Medicine
1400 Jackson Street
Denver, CO 80206
(800) 222–5864

Respiratory Nursing Society (RNS)
5700 Old Orchard Road, First Floor
Skokie, IL 60077–1057
(708) 966–8673

Internet Connections

Allergy, Asthma, and Immunology Online
Allergy LISTSERV List
Allergy and Asthma Network/Mothers of Asthmatics, Inc.
Alt.med.allergy Newsgroup
Alt.support.asthma Newsgroup
Alt.support.asthmaFAQ
Alt.support.non-smoker
American Academy of Allergy, Asthma, and Immunology (AAAAI) Web Site
AsmaNet
Asthma Zero Mortality Coalition (AZMC)
Asthma@infopro.com
Children's Mercy Hospital Allergy Home Page
International Food Information Council (IFIC) Foundation: Food Allergy
Johns Hopkins Office of Public Affairs, 76520–560@compuserve.com
Medical Reporter (a monthly on-line magazine)
MedLine
National Jewish Center for Immunology and Respiratory Medicine

National Institute of Allergy and Infectious Diseases
News from AAAI Meeting: Accolate for Asthma
On-Line Allergy Center (allergy@sig.net)
Pharmaceutical Information Network Home Page
U.S. Department of Health and Human Services
Warner-Lambert: Allergy-Cold-Cough-Sinus Medications
Weather-Health   Link   (http://www.inforamp.net/
   eeyore/asthma2.html)

Glossary

Adrenaline: See *epinephrine*.

Aerosol: A fine mist or spray of tiny particles. Many medications for respiratory diseases are in aerosol form and can be inhaled from a special, small pressurized can called a metered-dose inhaler. This sprays a controlled amount of the medicated mist through a mouth piece. Alternatively, the aerosol may be inhaled from an electric nebulizer.

Allergens: Substances that trigger the body's allergic reaction. When the IgE on a mast cell combines with an allergen, an allergic reaction may result.

Allergy: An overreaction of the immune system to an ordinarily harmless substance known as an allergen.

Anaphylaxis: The most severe form of allergy which can result in death if not treated immediately. This reaction involves the entire body with blood pressure's plunging to dangerously low levels, swelling throughout the body, hives, and airway collapse, so that the entry of air to the lungs is obstructed.

Antibiotics: Drugs that kill bacteria or slow down their reproduction. By doing this, they help the body's own immune defenses such as the white blood cells and various antibodies to clear bacteria from the body.

Antibodies: Specific types of proteins called immunoglobulins, which are part of the body's defense mechanism. Antibodies are made to neutralize a foreign protein in the body.

Apneas: Cessations of breathing which may occur during sleep. These apneas are ended by an audible resumption of breathing and continuation of snoring.

Autonomic nervous system: The system over which we have no voluntary control that regulates the organs in the body. It consists of two branches: the sympathetic and the parasympathetic nervous systems.

Alveoli: Tiny sacs that branch off the smallest airways like clusters of grapes.

Beta2-agonists: Powerful medications that may give quick relief for most cases of bronchospasm yet have no effect on the inflammation in the airway. Their primary action is to relax the muscle in the walls of the bronchial tubes.

Bronchi: The airways that connect the trachea (windpipe) to the lungs.

Bronchioles: The smaller airways in the lungs.

Bronchoconstriction: A narrowing of the bronchial airways which may cause wheezing or difficulty breathing.

Bronchoconstrictor: A substance that causes the airways in the lungs to narrow. Histamine is a bronchoconstrictor.

Bronchodilator: A drug that widens and relaxes the bronchi.

Bronchoscopy: A direct examination of the bronchial tubes.

Capillaries: Tiny blood vessels which carry blood for the pickup of oxygen from the freshly inhaled air in the alveoli.

Cell: The smallest living animal unit.

Central nervous system: The anatomical term for the brain and the spinal cord.

(COPD) chronic obstructive pulmonary disease: The term commonly used to describe four distinct problems: asthma, bronchiectasis, chronic bronchitis, and emphysema, all of which limit airflow.

Diaphragm: The muscle that separates the chest cavity from the abdomen. It is the main provider of inspiratory force and is called the second vital pump; the heart is considered the first.

Dyspnea: Shortness of breath, a feeling of breathlessness, or a sense of not getting enough air out of proportion to activity.

Epinephrine: A naturally occurring hormone that exerts important influences on the bronchial tubes, also called adrenaline. It helps keep the muscle in the walls of bronchi relaxed so the airway remains wide. It also suppresses the release of other substances, such as histamine, which cause mucus secretion and bronchospasm.

Eosinophils: A type of white blood cell associated with allergic diseases.

Extrinsic asthma: A type of asthma that develops at early age for those with a personal and family history of allergy. Other distinguishing features are increased numbers of certain white blood cells called *eosinophils*.

FEV-1: Forced expiratory volume in one second, or the amount of air forcefully exhaled in one second after filling the lungs with air during a deep inspiration.

Histamine: A substance in the body that causes nasal stuffiness and dripping in a cold or hay fever, bronchoconstriction in asthma, and itchy spots in a skin allergy.

Hormone: A chemical product of living cells that circulates in body fluids and produces a specific effect on the activity of cells in other parts of the body.

Hyperinflation: A condition that occurs when air becomes entrapped in the lungs.

Hiatus hernia: A protrusion of the stomach up through the diaphragm into the chest.

Immune system: Cells and proteins that work to protect the body from harmful, infectious microorganisms such as bacteria, viruses, and fungi.

Immunoglobulin E (IgE): The most important antibody during an allergic reaction. Everyone makes IgE; however, people who have a genetic predisposition toward allergy make larger quantities of this protective protein.

Immunotherapy: A form of allergy treatment to prevent reactions to pollens, dust mites, mold, insects, and animals. The person is given gradually increasing doses of the allergen or substance to which he or she is allergic to make the immune system less sensitive or reactive.

Intrinsic asthma: Usually begins in adulthood, exhibits little or no seasonal variation, and is not associated with allergies. The family history of asthma is also less important. Intrinsic asthma tends to worsen with age.

Lungs: The main part of the respiratory system that takes oxygen from the air into the bloodstream and allows carbon dioxide to escape from the body.

Mast cells: Allergy-causing cells in the mucous lining of the nose, sinuses, and bronchi. They contain chemicals like *histamine*.

Medulla: The part of the brain that receives and processes input related to changes in oxygen, carbon dioxide, and acid content in the blood.

Mitochondria: Minute structures within the cell where the oxidation of food takes place.

Mucokinetic agent: A drug that helps thin mucus to make it easier to flow.

Mucus: A viscid, slippery secretion produced by the mucous membrane, which helps to lubricate and protect certain parts of the body.

Mucous membrane: A soft, pink, skinlike structure that lines many cavities and tubes in the body, such as the respiratory tract. The mucous membrane secretes a fluid containing *mucus*.

NSAID: Nonsteroidal anti-inflammatory drug.

Oxidation: The combination of oxygen with the carbon and hydrogen atoms that make up food matter such as carbohydrates. During this process, energy is released that is used to drive the various life-supporting functions inside the cell.

Oxygen: An odorless, colorless gas that makes up 21 percent of the atmosphere on Earth. Oxygen is necessary for most forms of life and is absorbed through the lungs into the blood.

Parasympathetic nervous system: The part of the autonomic nervous system that produces acetylcholine in an asthma attack. This chemical stimulates the release of histamine, serotonin, and other chemical mediators from mast cells.

Pneumonia: An infection inside the lung associated with the collection of pus (white blood cells) in the alveoli and small bronchial tubes.

Pulmonary: Relating to the lungs.

Respiration: A basic process of life that enables us to have energy for growth and activity.

Rhonchi: Whistling or snoring sounds heard through the stethoscope when listening to the chest. Ronchi indicate partial obstruction of the airways by mucus or other inflammatory debris such as pus.

Sympathetic nervous system: The part of the autonomic nervous system that produces epinephrine in a response to stress. In an asthma attack, triggering the sympathetic branch causes airways to expand or dilate.

Trachea: The main airway which divides into large bronchial tubes going to each lung.

Triggers: The factors that cause an asthma attack by initiating airway inflammation and bronchospasm.

Turbinates: Tubular structures that project into the nasal chambers and increase the surface area of the walls inside the nose. A mucous membrane that is rich in blood vessels covers these turbinates. The turbinates may swell and cause nasal obstruction.

Vaccine: A preparation given to induce immunity against an infectious disease. Most vaccines contain weakened versions of the specific organisms against which immunity is sought. They do not cause the disease but stimulate the body's immune response to the infectious agent.

Vagus nerve: This nerve affects airway muscle tone and mucus secretion. When the vagus nerve is stimulated, acetylcholine, a chemical that contracts the airway muscle and causes mucus stimulation, is produced.

Wheeze: The sound heard during breathing that indicates an obstruction in the airways. It is usually heard during expiration but can sometimes be heard during inspiration.

Index